Homemade
Beauty

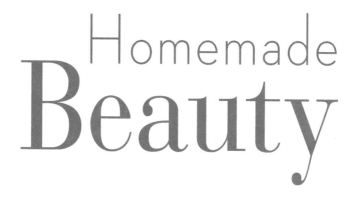

Homemade
Beauty

*150 Simple Beauty Recipes Made from
All-Natural Ingredients*

ANNIE STROLE

A PERIGEE BOOK

A PERIGEE BOOK
Published by the Penguin Group
Penguin Group (USA) LLC
375 Hudson Street, New York, New York 10014

USA • Canada • UK • Ireland • Australia • New Zealand • India • South Africa • China

penguin.com

A Penguin Random House Company

HOMEMADE BEAUTY

ISBN: 978-0-399-17102-4

An application to register this book for cataloging has been submitted to the Library of Congress.

First edition: December 2014

PRINTED IN THE UNITED STATES OF AMERICA

1   3   5   7   9   10   8   6   4   2

Text design by Ellen Cipriano
Illustrations by Rita Carroll

For Paul and Silas

Contents

INTRODUCTION   ix

Part One: Welcome to Homemade Beauty

Chapter 1: Why All-Natural Beauty Products?   3

Chapter 2: Ingredients   5

Chapter 3: Tools   8

Part Two: The Recipes

Chapter 4: Skin   13

   Cleansing Recipes   13

   Moisturizing Recipes   31

Detoxifying Recipes 43

Pampering Recipes 58

Chapter 5: Hair 73

Cleansing Recipes 73

Moisturizing Recipes 83

Detoxifying Recipes 101

Pampering Recipes 112

Chapter 6: Body 126

Cleansing Recipes 127

Moisturizing Recipes 135

Detoxifying Recipes 153

Pampering Recipes 160

RESOURCES 177

ACKNOWLEDGMENTS 183

INDEX 184

Introduction

Welcome to your guide to all-natural, toxin-free beauty products that you can create easily at home. This may sound daunting to some, but making your own products is one of the most empowering ways to take your beauty and health into your own hands. Just because the beauty products in stores contain tons of ingredients with extremely long and complicated names doesn't make all those chemicals necessary—don't let them overwhelm you. Making beauty products is a lot easier than you'd think.

Some of those ingredients can even be harmful. Pthalates, sodium lauryl and sodium laureth sulfate, propylene glycol, polyethylene glycol and the infamous parabens are just a few common beauty product ingredients that have been reported to cause irritation, cancer, organ abnormalities, hormone disruption and sterility.

Now that that's out of the way, for the majority of the book I want to focus on the enjoyable aspects of natural beauty rather than the disease-causing aspects of the unnatural variety. Handcrafting your own all-natural beauty products is extremely satisfying and fun. If you love DIY, then I'm certain that you'll enjoy creating some handmade beauty products. Additionally, making homemade beauty products is also a cost-effective and super thoughtful way of making gifts for friends and loved ones.

From the stance of a beauty professional, creating your own personalized homemade beauty products is a fantastic way to find solutions to problematic skin without blasting your face, hair and body with chemicals that may be detrimental down the line. I speak from experience.

After moving to New York from Texas, my skin had never looked worse. Stress, change of climate, change of water, pollution and who knows what else were clearly taking their toll, and my skin exacted its revenge with tons of huge, angry, inflamed zits. Of course, my first course of action was to evaluate my diet, up my water intake and be sure to be active and sleep well, but then I took a look at what I was putting on my skin. After some research I discovered my ordinary store-bought cleanser was mostly petroleum-based, preservative-filled garbage. I began researching more natural brands, and as I did that, I realized a lot of their active and most effective ingredients were those found in my kitchen. As a makeup artist and beauty addict, I'd always been interested in skin care, but once I embarked upon my natural skincare sleuthing, my interest turned to an obsession.

For my imbalanced, acned condition, a friend suggested I use raw apple cider vinegar as a toner after cleansing. I began seeing drastic improvement in my complexion, and started trusting all-natural ingredients to care for my skin. I also began using tea tree oil to zap away zits, and a lemon and honey concoction to decongest my pores (you can find the recipe for that in the Detoxifying section of the Skin chapter!). Day by day my skin was improving and eventually returned to a state of homeostasis.

I began to wonder what natural ingredients could do for my dry hair and body. Natural oils, fruits, yogurt and a number of other items found in my very own kitchen did a fantastic job of nourishing and hydrating my hair and skin. At this point I was hooked on educating myself about, and randomly slathering on, all types of edible ingredients.

Of course I had to spread the love, and I began posting a few recipes on Lovelyish.com, where I work as a contributing editor. I also started making all-natural recipe recommendations to friends, family and even clients. Through this process, not only did I educate others but I learned a great deal about how certain ingredients affect and benefit skin types other than mine (in addition to receiving quite a few recommendations myself).

The recipes that you'll find in this book are a collection of ones I happened upon myself, in addition to personal adaptations of recipes that were recommended to me. As you read this book and hand-craft your own products, I encourage you to be creative and trust your instincts to adapt these recipes to best fit your needs. You may notice that these recipes are translated in cups, tablespoons, drops, squeezes and handfuls—if you were mass-producing products for continuity or working with chemicals, this wouldn't fly. But that's the beauty of these recipes: Perfection isn't required. Sure, it may be ideal to create some of these products by measuring weight in ounces, but I'm assuming most of you don't have a kitchen scale at home (but if you do, fantastic!). A teaspoon over or ⅛ of a cup under what the recipe calls for certainly won't ruin your recipe . . . in fact, you may find that tweaking ingredients benefits your skin! Everyone's skin is different; therefore, what works for you might be completely different than what works for me. You have to experiment!

I hope you enjoy reading this book and creating your own beauty products as much as I enjoyed writing this guide. Don't be afraid to make messes and get your hands dirty in the name of beauty!

Icon Key

Throughout the book you'll notice a number of icons intended to guide you to the homemade beauty product best suited for yourself or the recipient of your product in addition to informing you as to whether or not the product is suited for only one use or can be stored or made in batches. Be sure to look out for the following icons!

ICON KEY

GENERAL:

🎁 makes a great gift

① for one-time use only

SKIN:

⬥ suitable for all skin types

⬥ suitable for all skin types except sensitive

⬥ suitable for normal to dry skin

⬥ suitable for normal to oily skin

⬥ suitable for oily, acne-prone skin

⬥ suitable for mature skin

HAIR:

● suitable for all hair types

● suitable for normal to oily hair

● suitable for normal to dry hair

● suitable for dry hair

● suitable for fine hair

BODY:

◼ suitable for all skin types

◼ suitable for normal skin

◼ suitable for normal to dry skin

PART ONE

Welcome to Homemade Beauty

chapter 1

Why All-Natural Beauty Products?

By now, it's clear that eating a diet that consists mostly of organic fruits and vegetables is most beneficial to our health, but what about caring for our largest organ and our first line of defense: our skin?

You may be washing your face every night, using moisturizer, eye cream and sunscreen and treating yourself to masks and exfoliants, but if the products you're using are jam-packed with toxic chemicals and preservatives, you're probably not doing yourself too many favors.

It turns out that ingredients such as sulfates, parabens and artificial fragrances that have commonly been used in skin-, hair- and body-care products for decades are now being found to cause inflammatory skin reactions and are even suspected to cause some serious diseases, illnesses and hormonal issues with extended use. Other ingredients like additives and fillers simply suffocate the skin and are a waste of money.

Just like our bodies benefit from eating fresh, natural, unprocessed foods, our skin thrives when we treat it with the same quality ingredients. You'll be surprised when you notice the effects that a natural treatment has on your skin after the first use. While there are some fabulous (and expensive!) all-natural skincare products on the market, there's no denying that making fresh products in your own home is more beneficial. The recipes in this book are easy and fun and will greatly improve your skin, wallet and health.

chapter 2

Ingredients

· ·

The ingredients required for these recipes are not particularly out of the ordinary. For the most part we'll be using items (mostly fruits, vegetables and typical cooking ingredients) you may already have in your kitchen!

Just like I would suggest that you select high-quality, organic produce for your diet, I recommend the same for your beauty recipes. Don't worry: The recipes call for small amounts, so you'll have plenty of produce left over for meals or additional recipes. (I also really enjoy snacking on my ingredients as I make products . . . it's a win-win!)

There are certain recipes that require some specialty items such as beeswax, shea butter and other not-so-common supermarket finds, but these can easily be found at craft stores, health-food stores or online. Amazon.com is a veritable treasure trove of DIY beauty supplies, and Mountainroseherbs.com has tons of high-quality essential oils, among many other specialty beauty items. I love NOW Solutions for its wide variety of high-quality carrier oils, which can be found in health-food stores or online.

As far as castile soap, an extremely gentle oil-based soap that you'll see mentioned in a number of recipes, I love Dr. Bronner's Unscented Baby-Mild Castile Soap, but you can find a variety of brands online or at your local health-food store, and even at many grocery or beauty-supply stores.

Again, just as you would if you were eating it, be sure to wash all produce required in recipes and check that any other food-grade items are not past their expiration date—this can drastically affect the outcome of your recipes!

Specifics on Recommended Ingredients

- Coconut oil—unrefined virgin (Nutiva is my personal favorite brand)
- Olive oil—extra-virgin
- Apple cider vinegar—raw, organic (Bragg is my favorite brand)
- Castile soap—Dr. Bronner's Unscented Baby-Mild Castile Soap
- Yogurt—always use plain yogurt. I prefer any type of Greek yogurt, but as long as it is plain and has active cultures, it will be effective.
- Honey—raw, organic honey is best and can be found

at your local health-food store or farmers market. Most regular honeys are cut with corn syrup, which won't do your skin any favors. Even better is if you can get your hands on some local honey, which helps support your area's beehives and has countless health and skin benefits (swallowing a tablespoon of the stuff daily will enormously ease pollen allergies!). I definitely recommend purchasing liquid raw honey, as opposed to the solid kind. It's much easier to work with, but both will do—you'll just have to be sure to melt your solid honey before including it in any of the recipes.

- Tea tree oil—a lot of tea tree oils are sold as blends, so be sure you purchase 100 percent tea tree oil.
- Shea butter—raw, unrefined (I purchase from Amazon and other online retailers)
- Cocoa butter—raw (also purchased from Amazon and other online retailers)
- Beeswax—pure, yellow. I prefer working with pellets so that you don't have to shave or chop a big block (and pellets are a lot easier to work with). I also purchase this from Amazon and other online retailers.
- Vegetable glycerine—can be found on Amazon, at health-food stores or at other online retailers

chapter 3

Tools

....

Homemade Beauty **is about** being simple and approachable; just like the ingredients are mostly commonplace, the tools aren't intimidating, either. The utensils required are not dissimilar to those you would need for cooking or baking. You probably already own most of them!

Measuring cups and spoons

Saucepan

Double boiler (or a Pyrex measuring cup in a pot of boiling water works just as well)

Blender or food processor

Hand mixer

Cutlery (fork, spoon and knife)

Cutting board
Bowls (small to medium)
Containers (small jars, bottles, squeeze bottles and
    spray bottles)
A sifter
Small funnel
Soap molds (can be purchased from craft stores, at
    Amazon.com or at other online retailers)
Juicer*

---

* Required for only one recipe in this book.

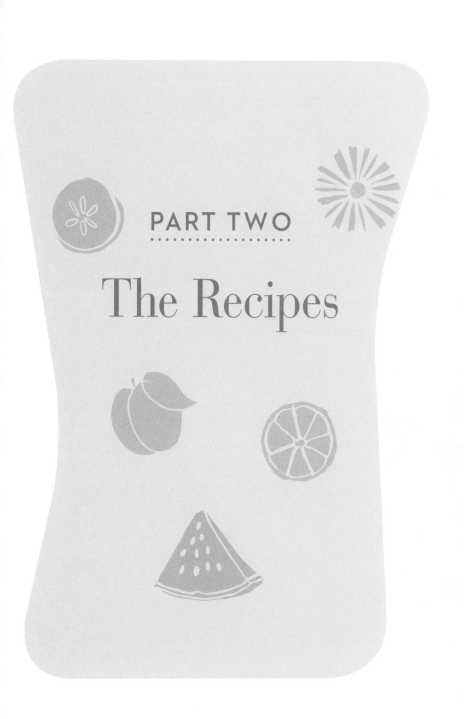

PART TWO

The Recipes

chapter 4

Skin

∙ ∙

From cleansers and toners to moisturizers and masks, the recipes found in this chapter are intended to address any skincare concerns—whether it's acne, wrinkles, dehydration or just the maintenance of beautiful skin, using all-natural means.

My face was the first area I began experimenting with with all-natural homemade products, so this section holds a special place in my heart. If my incredibly problematic skin was able to benefit from just a few food-grade concoctions, then anyone's can.

Cleansing Recipes

These recipes are intended to remove dirt and residue from the face. If you wear makeup, it is imperative that you remove it before cleansing . . . or you could just use the first recipe of this section, which is a two-in-one makeup-removing cleanser! What's great about all-natural cleansers is that you can create one that is incredibly effective without harming the homeostasis of your delicate facial skin—unlike many of the harsh and stripping or petroleum-filled and ineffective cleansers on the market!

The cleansing oils and toners of this section can make great gifts, but most of these cleansers are intended for one-time use only.

Olive Oil–Rose Makeup-Removing Cleanser

½ cup distilled water

¼ cup rose water

1 teaspoon liquid castile soap

1 tablespoon extra-virgin olive oil

This soothing, makeup-dissolving face wash thoroughly cleanses your skin while leaving it feeling hydrated and pampered. Olive oil actively removes makeup and debris, and rose water continuously cleanses, refreshes and hydrates.

Combine all ingredients in a small bottle and shake gently. For use, wet face with warm water, work cleanser between hands to create a lather, massage all over face and rinse thoroughly.

All-Natural Makeup-Removing Wipes

1 paper towel roll, cut in half (You'll want to do this
    with a large serrated knife. Leave the paper
    towels on the roll and "saw" them in half,
    creating two short paper towel rolls. Remove
    the cardboard tube.)
1 small, round resealable plastic container that will
    fit the width of the paper towel roll
2 cups distilled water
1 tablespoon unrefined virgin coconut oil
1 tablespoon jojoba oil
1 teaspoon vitamin E oil

There's no denying the ease and convenience of makeup-removing wipes, but most brands on the market contain lots of unsavory ingredients, and I've bought plenty that don't even remove makeup very well! Making your own makeup-removing wipes is an incredibly fun craft that also provides you with the peace of mind that your product contains zero harmful chemicals—and these totally pulverize any stubborn mascara or liner.

Melt coconut oil in double boiler or until liquefied (about 15 to 25 seconds) in the microwave. (If you don't have a double boiler, you can simply combine the two ingredients in a Pyrex measuring cup and then place it in a saucepan containing a small amount of water and heat until the wax liquefies.) Pour coconut oil and all liquid ingredients into resealable plastic container. Place the lid on the container and shake to combine ingredients.

Open the container and place one half roll of paper towels inside, allowing the paper towels to soak up the liquid. It may need to "marinate" for 5 to 10 minutes to allow the roll to become completely soaked.

Once the roll is completely soaked, push it down so it fits entirely in the container. Place lid on the container and store in a cool, dry place.

To use, wipe dry face with wet wipes, concentrating on the areas with the most makeup application. Rinse or follow with a cleanser if necessary.

Olive Oil Eye-Makeup Remover

2 tablespoons extra-virgin olive oil
1 teaspoon liquid castile soap
$\frac{1}{4}$ cup distilled water

Olive oil is incredible for sweeping away stubborn eye makeup in seconds while keeping the delicate eye area hydrated. This recipe makes a better eye-makeup remover than anything on the market that I've tried!

Combine ingredients in a small bottle. Be sure to shake thoroughly before each use. To use, apply a small amount to a cotton ball or pad and gently sweep away eye makeup.

Vitamin E Oil

Vitamin E oil is an ingredient that you see a lot of in this book, and for good reason. Not only does it plump skin, reduce scarring and lighten brown spots, but it also is full of antioxidants. These antioxidants obviously benefit the skin by fighting free radicals, but they also work to prolong the shelf life of your homemade ingredients. You'll notice that only small amounts of the oil is used—too much vitamin E oil can be heavy and aggravate breakouts, so you always want to use it sparingly.

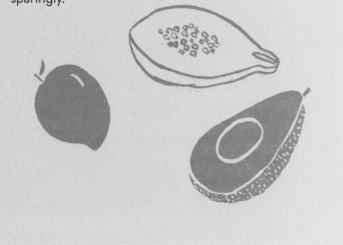

Personalized Facial Cleansing Oil

FOR NORMAL SKIN:

2 tablespoons sunflower seed oil

2 tablespoons castor oil

FOR OILY SKIN:

1 tablespoon jojoba oil

2 tablespoons castor oil

If you are also acne-prone, add in 5 drops of tea tree oil.

FOR COMBINATION SKIN:

2 tablespoons sweet almond oil

2 tablespoons castor oil

FOR DRY SKIN:

2 tablespoons avocado oil

1 tablespoon castor oil

As a longtime sufferer of acne-prone oily skin, the thought of intentionally slathering oil on my face made me cringe. Finally, I worked up the guts to try it, and I've never looked back. It turns out that applying noncomedogenic oils to your face actually balances the oil level in your skin, which stops it from overproducing oil and instead leaves it even and clear. Different skin types require different oils, although all cleansing oils should contain castor oil, as it provides antiseptic qualities.

Combine the oils specified for your skin type in a small bottle and shake gently to blend.

To use, apply 1 teaspoon of blended oil to face and massage thoroughly for 1 to 2 minutes. Use a warm washcloth to thoroughly wipe excess oil from your skin.

If your skin feels tight or dry after cleansing, pat a few drops of the cleansing oil on your face for added moisture.

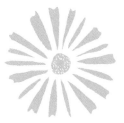

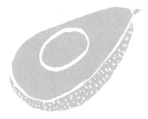

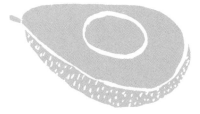

Soothing Lavender-Rose Water Toner

1 cup rose water
1 teaspoon vegetable glycerine
6 drops lavender essential oil

Toners are fantastic for providing an additional cleanse, as well as helping to balance and moisturize the skin. This formulation is light-weight, hydrating and calming, so it's perfect if your skin is dry and sensitive.

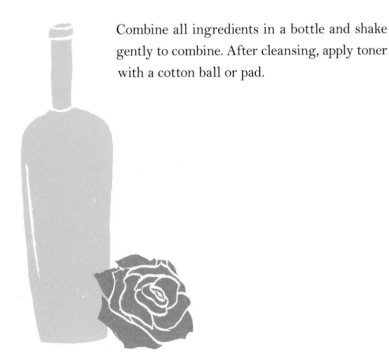

Combine all ingredients in a bottle and shake gently to combine. After cleansing, apply toner with a cotton ball or pad.

Oatmeal-Yogurt Cleanser

1 cup rolled oats
½ cup plain yogurt

Oatmeal is a skincare superhero: It soothes, hydrates, exfoliates and balances the skin. Pair it with yogurt and you can create an amazing exfoliating and hydrating cleanser, or leave it on for 5 to 10 minutes as a mask!

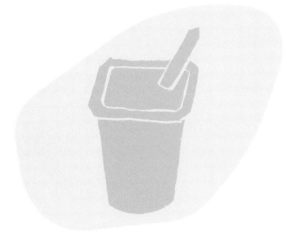

Mix ingredients in a bowl to create a paste. Gently massage cleanser all over face and either let sit for the time indicated above as a mask or rinse thoroughly.

Apple Cider Vinegar Toner

1 cup distilled water
½ cup apple cider vinegar

Apple cider vinegar is an incredible ingredient not only in the kitchen but for your beauty cabinet as well. This toner will balance the pH of your skin, in addition to sloughing off dead skin cells and helping to fade the appearance of scars.

Combine ingredients in resealable container of your choice. Shake well before each use, and apply after cleansing with a cotton ball or pad. Mix up a new batch once a month.

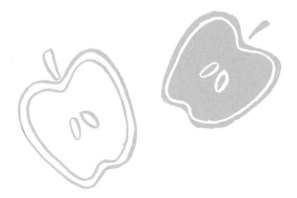

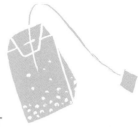

Tea Tree-Basil Anti-Acne Toner

1½ cups distilled water
3 tablespoons dried basil leaves
6 drops tea tree essential oil

Basil is more commonly known as a kitchen herb, but it works wonders for acne-prone skin, acting as a natural, gentle antiseptic. Tea tree oil is widely used for its antibacterial benefits.

Bring water to a boil, and allow the basil to steep (either in a tea ball or loose, however you prefer), like you would a tea, for up to 2 hours. Once the mixture is cool, if you have left the basil loose while steeping, strain out and add tea tree oil. Store in a bottle or jar, and apply with a cotton ball or pad after cleansing.

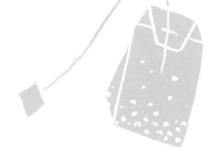

Brightening Citrus Toner

1½ cups distilled water
Zest of 1 lemon
Zest of 1 orange
Juice of 1 lemon
3 drops tangerine essential oil (optional)

Citrus is extremely invigorating, and the vitamin C it contains helps to brighten skin while fading discoloration. I love storing this toner in a spray bottle in the fridge and using it as a refreshing mist. Adding tangerine essential oil is also great because it adds to the citrusy fragrance, has antibacterial properties and creates a calming aura.

Bring water to a boil, remove from heat and combine in a glass jar with the lemon and orange zests. Let mixture steep overnight in the refrigerator. Strain out the zest, pour product into resealable container of your choice and squeeze in the fresh lemon juice. Add tangerine oil, if desired, and apply with a cotton ball or spray bottle.

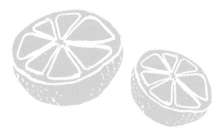

Detoxifying Green Tea Toner

1½ cups water
4 bags green tea
Juice of 1 lemon

Drinking a cup of green tea a day is sure to make you feel like a new person, so treating your face topically with green tea can totally transform your skin. Green tea detoxifies from the inside out and the outside in! This toner is great for clogged, congested pores and is incredibly refreshing.

Bring water to a boil and steep the tea bags for up to 2 hours in the fridge. After steeping, remove tea bags and add freshly squeezed lemon juice. Pour into resealable container of your choice and sweep on with a cotton ball after cleansing.

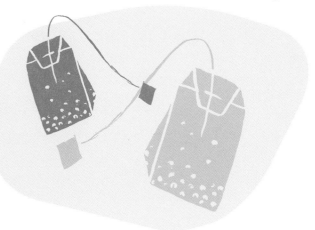

Refreshing Cucumber Toner

½ cucumber, finely chopped
¼ cup rose water
1 teaspoon vegetable glycerine

This is another great toner for keeping in the fridge for a refreshing, extremely hydrating pick-me-up! Cucumber and rose water refresh, soothe and add moisture to the skin without being oily or overwhelming.

Add ingredients to a blender and blend on high until smooth. Strain liquid into resealable container of your choice. Apply with a cotton ball or keep it in a spray bottle for a beautifying mist! Store at room temperature or in the fridge for optimal effects.

Brightening and Exfoliating Strawberry Mask

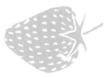

6 strawberries
1 tablespoon yogurt
1 teaspoon honey

Strawberries are jam-packed with vitamin C and plenty of other skin-loving antioxidants. They also contain a gentle acid that exfoliates, brightens skin and fades dark spots. This mask is great for dull skin and also happens to make a delicious snack.

Place ingredients in a blender or food processor and blend on low until smooth. Spread the mask evenly over face, and let sit for 20 minutes. Rinse thoroughly with warm water.

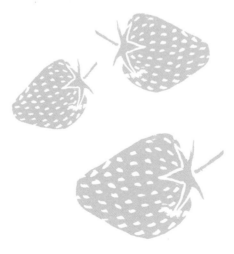

Oatmeal-Chocolate Exfoliating Face Treatment

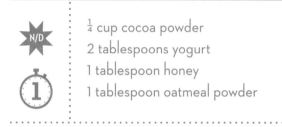

¼ cup cocoa powder
2 tablespoons yogurt
1 tablespoon honey
1 tablespoon oatmeal powder

This indulgent mask employs the powerful antioxidants of cocoa and the soothing, exfoliating capabilities of oatmeal. This recipe calls for oatmeal powder, but you could also just grind an equal amount of rolled oats in your food processor.

Stir all ingredients in a bowl, blending thoroughly. Quickly spread the mask evenly over face, as this recipe tends to harden a bit. Leave on for 20 minutes, and rinse thoroughly with warm water.

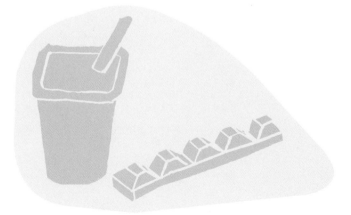

Exfoliating Papaya Peel

1 papaya, peeled, deseeded and chopped
1 tablespoon honey
Juice of 1 lemon

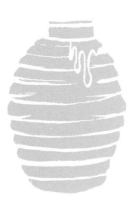

Papayas are incredible for topical use due to their healing and exfoliating enzymes, which act similar to alpha hydroxy acid. This mask reduces fine lines, moisturizes and gives skin a beautiful glow.

Place the papaya in a blender and blend on high until the fruit is smooth and pastelike. Pour it into a bowl and stir in honey and freshly squeezed lemon juice. This mask tends to be thin, so you may want to apply it with a clean foundation brush. Leave on for 15 minutes and rinse thoroughly with warm water.

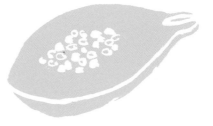

Brightening Lemon Cleanser

½ cup liquid castile soap
¼ cup distilled water
Juice of ½ lemon
1 teaspoon vitamin E oil

Over time, continued use of this cleanser will bring about evenly toned skin and a marked reduction in blackheads. Achieving brighter and less congested skin can be as easy as using this simple lemon juice cleanser twice a day.

Combine castile soap and water in the face wash container (I personally prefer squeeze-top containers). Squeeze in lemon juice through a strainer to catch any pulp or seeds. Add vitamin E oil and shake to combine. Shake before each use.

Moisturizing Recipes

Beautiful skin is moisturized skin; even if your skin is oily, it is imperative to keep it hydrated. Moisture can prevent or reduce the appearance of wrinkles and can help heal any scars or blemishes. The recipes found here are hydrating oils, lotions, creams, treatments and masks, so you're sure to find one best suited for your skin type!

Orange Creamsicle Mask

$\frac{1}{4}$ cup yogurt
1 tablespoon honey
Juice of 1 orange
3 drops tangerine essential oil

This supremely hydrating mask is perfect for those days that nothing you seem to be putting on your face is moisturizing enough. The vitamin C of the orange will remove dead skin cells, allowing the hydrating yogurt to penetrate the skin.

Stir ingredients together in a small bowl until a consistent paste forms. Spread all over face and leave on for 20 minutes. Rinse thoroughly with warm water.

Olive Oil and Honey Mask

1 teaspoon extra-virgin olive oil
1 tablespoon honey

Achieving instant hydration could not be any easier! Honey is a fantastic moisturizer, and olive oil deeply penetrates, plumps and nourishes the skin. This mask is so gentle it can be used every day, but even used once a week, you'll notice more youthful, hydrated skin.

Stir your ingredients together until thoroughly blended. Pat mask on until it becomes tacky. (This ensures that the mask thoroughly penetrates and stimulates your skin.) Leave on for 10 minutes. Rinse thoroughly with warm water.

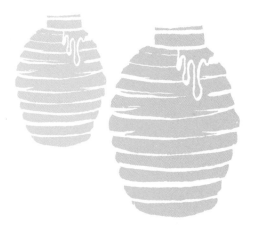

Revitalizing Cucumber-Avocado Mask

$\frac{1}{4}$ cucumber, chopped
1 avocado, stoned and
   peeled
1 tablespoon yogurt
1 teaspoon honey

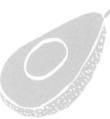

Cooling cucumber and nutrient-rich avocado combine to make a super-refreshing and moisturizing mask for dehydrated, dull skin. This is also a great treatment to use if you're just feeling overheated and in need of a pick-me-up!

Place ingredients in a blender and blend on low or medium until smooth. Apply mask and let sit for 20 minutes. For a full-on spa-treatment effect, slice remaining cucumber and use two pieces as eye pads! Rinse thoroughly with warm water.

Hydrating Watermelon Mask

1 cup watermelon, cubed
1 tablespoon yogurt
1 teaspoon honey

It's pretty obvious that watermelon is hydrating; it is 93 percent water, after all. But did you know that it's also jam-packed with antioxidants, vitamins and minerals? It's the ultimate skincare fruit. This mask is a wonderful, refreshing treat that can be used as often as you like! Watermelons can be really daunting to cut, so I like to take it easy on myself and buy the pre-cut version from the grocery store. Is that cheating?

Place ingredients in a blender and blend until smooth. Spread evenly over face and leave on for 20 minutes. Rinse thoroughly with warm water.

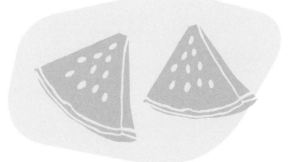

Shea and Cocoa Butter
Intense Hydrating Face Cream

$\frac{1}{4}$ cup shea butter

$\frac{1}{4}$ cup cocoa butter

$\frac{1}{4}$ cup extra-virgin olive oil

$\frac{1}{4}$ cup unrefined virgin coconut oil

This recipe not only creates the most hydrating, protective and pampering face cream ever, but it also is extremely fun to make. This recipe keeps for quite some time, so it can make a great DIY gift.

Melt the shea and cocoa butter and coconut oil in a double boiler and remove from heat. Let cool for a half hour. Stir in olive oil and the essential oil of your choice. Chill your ingredients in the fridge until they partially solidify, and then whip with a hand mixer until a creamy consistency is achieved. Package in a glass jar and apply after cleansing and toning.

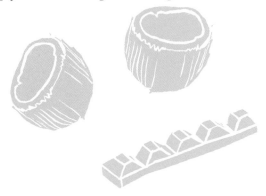

Soothing Chamomile and Oatmeal Face Treatment

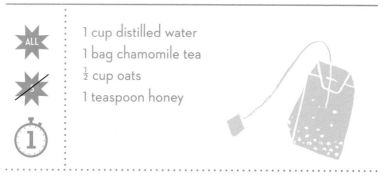

1 cup distilled water
1 bag chamomile tea
$\frac{1}{2}$ cup oats
1 teaspoon honey

Soothe, exfoliate and hydrate with this straight-from-the-spa treatment. Chamomile instantly eliminates redness and comforts the skin while oatmeal continuously calms and diminishes dead skin cells.

Bring water to a boil and steep tea bag for 5 minutes. Slowly pour hot tea into the oats until a thick paste is formed. Let this sit for 5 minutes. If the paste is still too thick, add a small amount of tea until the desired consistency is reached. Stir in the honey and blend your treatment thoroughly.

Gently massage chamomile oatmeal treatment onto clean face and neck using circular motions. Manipulate the product for 1 to 2 minutes, and then rinse thoroughly with warm water.

Lavender Lip Balm

1½ tablespoons beeswax
1 tablespoon cocoa butter
1 tablespoon unrefined virgin coconut oil
1 tablespoon sweet almond oil
4 drops vitamin E oil
10 drops vanilla oil
5 drops lavender essential oil

Lip balm is a product most of us can't (and shouldn't) do without. Who would have thought that you could make the most hydrating and healthiest lip balm in your own home? This recipe has a long shelf life and can make a beautiful gift.

In a double boiler, melt beeswax, cocoa butter and coconut oil. Once melted, remove ingredients from heat and stir in the remaining oils. Pour the liquid into your desired lip balm packaging (I recommend a small glass jar or stainless steel tin) and let cool for a half hour before putting the lid on the container.

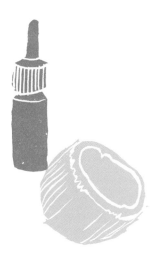

Honey-Cocoa Butter Lip Balm

1½ tablespoons beeswax
1 tablespoon cocoa butter
1 tablespoon shea butter
1 teaspoon raw organic honey
10 drops vanilla oil

This lip balm is so delicious you'll want to eat it! Luckily, since the ingredients are all natural, you could if you wanted to, although I don't recommend it. This recipe would make the perfect holiday gift.

Melt beeswax and cocoa and shea butters in a double boiler. After ingredients have melted, remove from heat and slowly drizzle honey in while stirring thoroughly. Stir in vanilla oil. Pour liquid into your lip balm container and let it sit for a half hour before putting on the lid.

Skin-Tightening Egg White Mask

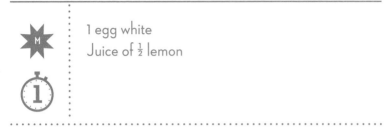

1 egg white
Juice of ½ lemon

Egg whites are a natural astringent that work to tighten and tone the skin. This recipe may be a little daring for those afraid to slather raw egg on their face, but I promise the results are worth it!

Whisk ingredients together until blended and the egg white becomes foamy. Apply mask, evenly covering face, especially the jawline. Let sit for 10 minutes, and rinse with warm water.

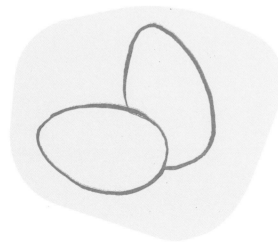

Firming Peach Mask

1 peach, pitted and chopped
1 tablespoon yogurt
1 teaspoon honey

When applied topically, peaches work to support the collagen in skin, in addition to being supremely hydrating. As an added bonus, peach gently unclogs pores! The yogurt exfoliates and hydrates while honey continuously moisturizes.

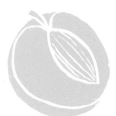

Place ingredients in a blender and blend on low or medium until smooth. Apply mask evenly to face, and let sit for 20 minutes. Rinse thoroughly with warm water.

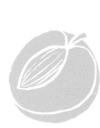
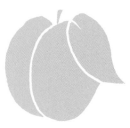

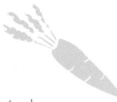

Carrot-Avocado Anti-Aging Mask

½ large carrot, chopped
½ avocado
1 tablespoon honey

This recipe makes the ultimate anti-aging mask. The nutrients in carrots and avocados help build collagen and elastin, moisturize and even eliminate age spots! Use this mask once or twice a week for best results.

Bring a medium saucepan of water to a boil. Cook carrot for approximately 10 to 15 minutes, until soft. Drain, mash into a paste-like consistency and let cool. Chop and mash avocado until smooth. Combine carrot and avocado with honey, and apply mixture evenly over face. Let sit for 20 minutes, and rinse thoroughly with warm water.

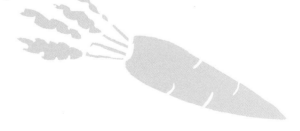

Soothing Lavender Eye Balm

1 tablespoon beeswax
1 tablespoon shea butter
1 tablespoon cocoa butter
1 tablespoon unrefined virgin coconut oil
1 tablespoon avocado oil
5 drops lavender essential oil
5 drops jasmine essential oil
2 drops patchouli essential oil

During winter months or when experiencing allergies, many of us deal with a dry, flaky, irritated under-eye area, and under-eye creams don't seem to cut it. This super-luxurious eye balm instantly diminishes flakiness, soothes the delicate skin under the eye and combats darkness and aging.

Melt beeswax, shea butter, cocoa butter and coconut oil in a double boiler. After melting, remove from heat, and stir in remaining oils until thoroughly blended. Pour liquid into a resealable small glass jar, and let cool with the container open before securing the lid.

Apply to clean eye area at night.

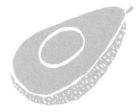

Balancing Face Oil

2 tablespoons grapeseed oil
2 tablespoons jojoba oil

You may think I'm totally crazy for recommending oils for oily skin, but oils have been an absolute lifesaver for my oily, acne-prone and acne-scarred face. Oils work to balance face oil by telling your skin to stop overproducing sebum. A good many oils are surprisingly lightweight and give just the right amount of hydration to oily faces. In fact, if your skin is oily or acne-prone, I recommend this recipe for hydrating over all the others in this chapter. The following recipe is perfect for healing, balancing and hydrating oily skin.

Combine oils in a small dropper bottle, and pat on 2 to 3 drops morning and night after cleansing.

After a few weeks, you'll notice your skin become less oily and clogged.

Detoxifying Recipes

If your skin is looking sallow, dull or congested (meaning full of blackheads and clogged pores), it's time to do some serious detoxifying. First, up your water intake, and then try a few of these detoxifying treatments according to your skin type!

Decongesting Pineapple Treatment

1 cup pineapple, chopped

$\frac{1}{2}$ cup yogurt

1 teaspoon white sugar

Pineapples contain an enzyme called bromelain, which works wonders for eliminating dead skin cells and, in turn, decongesting clogged pores. This mask is perfect for those with adult acne—you want to be using enzymatic exfoliation, not harsh scrubs or chemicals, on your delicate skin. Use this mask once a week, and you'll see a dramatic difference in the texture and tone of your skin! Unless you are really handy with a knife, I definitely recommend buying pre-cut pineapples from the grocery store. Just make sure they're fresh!

Place pineapple and yogurt in a blender and blend until smooth. Transfer mixture to a bowl and stir in sugar. Gently massage treatment all over face, avoiding the eye area, for 1 to 2 minutes. Rinse with warm water.

Pineapple

I was certainly pleased to discover that my all-time favorite fruit is awesome for topical use on the skin. Packed with vitamins A and C and a plethora of B vitamins, pineapple also contains enzymes (specifically, bromelain) that dissolve dead skin cells and slow the aging process.

Anti-Aging Pumpkin Puree Mask

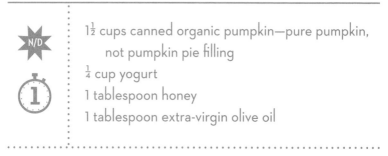

1½ cups canned organic pumpkin—pure pumpkin, not pumpkin pie filling

¼ cup yogurt

1 tablespoon honey

1 tablespoon extra-virgin olive oil

Pumpkins are another enzyme-packed food with skin-saving vitamins such as vitamins A, C and E. Used once or twice a week, this mask will remove dead skin cells while reducing fine lines and discoloration.

Stir ingredients together in a bowl and apply to clean skin. Let sit for 10 minutes. Wipe away any excess mask with a washcloth. Rinse thoroughly with warm water.

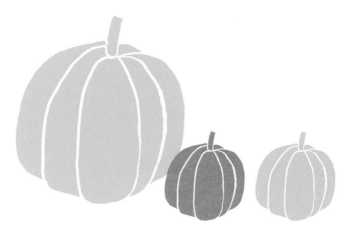

Supergreen Detox Smoothie Facial

½ cup fresh kale
¼ cup plain yogurt
1 tablespoon honey
Distilled water, as necessary

By now we all know the benefits of kale for our health, but the leafy green is also great for detoxifying and beautifying skin. Kale is rich in vitamin K, which helps reduce any darkness on the skin (if you have dark circles, you'll definitely want to apply this under your eyes, but be sure to avoid getting it too close to the eyes themselves), and it also contains tons of vitamin C, which helps the skin to fight free radicals and aids in collagen production. The lactic acid in yogurt gently exfoliates, allowing kale's nutrients to penetrate the skin more effectively.

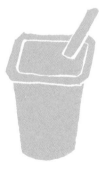

Place ingredients in a blender, and blend on high speed until thoroughly combined. If mixture is too thick, add small amounts of distilled water to reach desired consistency (you want a medium thickness, but nothing too soupy).

Apply to clean, dry skin, and allow to sit for 15 minutes. Rinse thoroughly, and follow with moisturizer.

Oil-Reducing Banana Mask

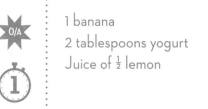

1 banana
2 tablespoons yogurt
Juice of ½ lemon

Banana works to reduce oil, acne and pore size while maintaining moisture and giving skin a beautiful glow. Use this mask twice a week, and you'll notice a dramatic difference in your skin.

Mash banana until free of lumps. Transfer to a bowl and stir in yogurt and lemon juice. Apply evenly over face, focusing on your T-zone (your forehead, nose and chin), where oil is most prevalent. Let sit for 20 minutes, and rinse thoroughly with warm water.

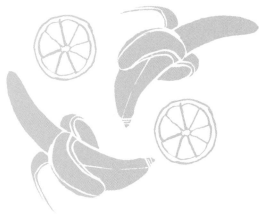

Anti-Acne Baking Soda Mask

2 tablespoons baking soda
2 tablespoons distilled water
4 to 5 drops lemon juice

If you're looking for an easy, inexpensive and all-natural way to combat acne, you will especially love this recipe. It doesn't get any more simple than this! Baking soda opens pores and eliminates the top layer of skin while lemon juice detoxifies and decongests. Use once a week.

Combine baking soda with water until a paste forms. Stir in drops of lemon juice and apply over affected area. Leave on for 5 to 10 minutes, and rinse thoroughly with water.

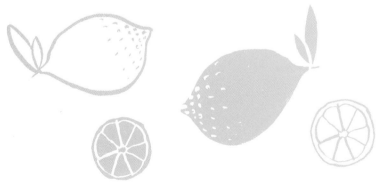

Tea Tree Zit Eraser

1 tablespoon tea tree essential oil
3 tablespoons jojoba oil

Tea tree's antibacterial properties work wonders for reducing zits. Jojoba oil most closely resembles the face's natural oil, so when applied topically it tells your face to stop producing oil. Combine these two together, and you have a serious acne-zapping spot treatment! This zit eraser gets rid of blemishes and keeps them from coming back.

Combine ingredients in a small bottle and shake well. Apply to clean skin nightly with a Q-tip or a clean finger until blemishes disappear.

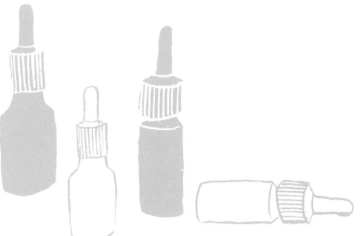

Lemon and Honey Blackhead Eraser

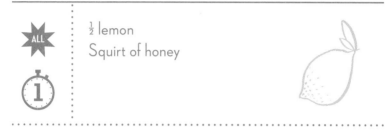

½ lemon
Squirt of honey

Blackheads are probably one of the most frustrating skincare dilemmas. Try all you want to get rid of them, but these pesky little clogged pores are often caused by things we can hardly control, like our environment and sebum production. Luckily, there is an all-natural, farm-fresh way to keep blackheads at bay!

Squirt honey on the exposed flesh of lemon, then rub the mixture over affected areas. Let sit for 10 minutes, and rinse.

Repeat this process once or twice a week and you'll see a dramatic reduction in blackheads.

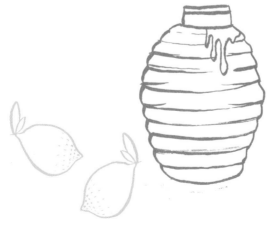

Detoxifying Blueberry-Yogurt Mask

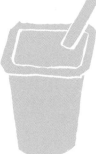

½ cup blueberries
2 tablespoons yogurt
Handful of raw almonds, chopped
Juice of ½ lemon

You know when your skin is breaking out, congested or just downright dull that it's time to do a little detoxifying! This antioxidant-packed recipe is as delicious as it is beautifying. It's super fun to make, spread on your face and even sample a taste of!

Place all ingredients in blender, and blend on high speed until smooth. Spread the mask evenly over face, and let it sit for 20 minutes. Rinse thoroughly.

Yogurt

Plain old yogurt: Sounds boring, but it is actually one of the most incredible things you can put in your hair and on your skin. It contains lactic acid, which gently exfoliates and hydrates the skin, not to mention all of yogurt's wonderful live cultures, which help balance skin and hair to give it a beautiful glow.

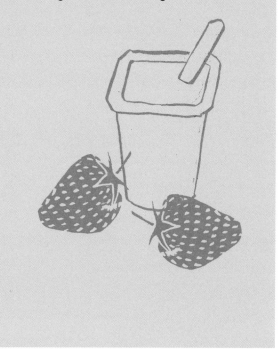

Lemon-Yogurt
Dark Spot–Lightening Treatment

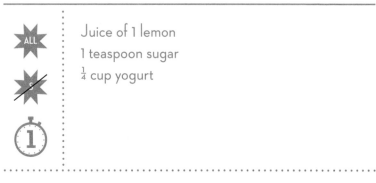

Juice of 1 lemon

1 teaspoon sugar

$\frac{1}{4}$ cup yogurt

The vitamin C in lemons drastically reduces dark spots and lightens discoloration but tends to be drying when used on its own. Combine it with moisturizing yogurt, and you have the perfect dark spot–lightening treatment.

Place lemon juice in a small bowl, add sugar and let stand for 5 minutes. Stir yogurt into juice, and combine thoroughly. Apply treatment to affected areas, and let sit for 20 minutes. Rinse with warm water, and be sure to moisturize afterward.

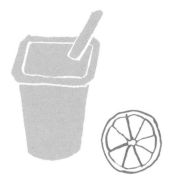

Acne Scar Eraser

1 teaspoon nutmeg
1 tablespoon honey

The only thing more frustrating than acne is the scarring that it often leaves behind. It takes about as much concealer to cover up acne scars as it does to cover the actual zit! Get even with acne scars with this awesome and super-simple acne scar eraser. Both honey and nutmeg are antifungal and anti-inflammatory, thus healing scars faster than ever.

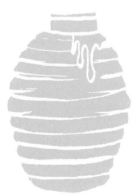

Combine ingredients and apply to affected area. Allow to sit for at least 30 minutes. Rinse thoroughly, and cleanse, if desired.

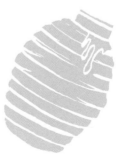

Detoxifying Clay Mask

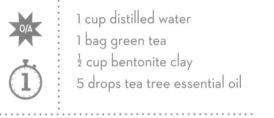

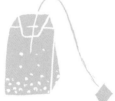

1 cup distilled water
1 bag green tea
½ cup bentonite clay
5 drops tea tree essential oil

Clay is the most powerful ingredient available to combat congested pores; at the same time, clay is completely safe and gentle. That said, this mask is very strong and extremely effective—your skin will feel very tight—so you want to make sure to moisturize after use!

Boil water and steep tea bag for 2 minutes. Allow the tea to cool, and then combine it with bentonite clay and tea tree oil. Apply all over face, concentrating on congested areas. Let sit for 30 minutes, and rinse with hot water; then splash with cold water.

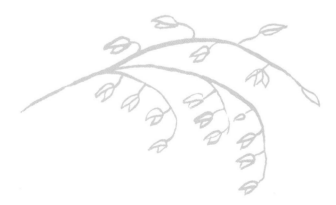

Detoxifying Herbal Acne Steam

¼ cup fresh basil

¼ cup fresh rosemary

¼ cup fresh peppermint

10 drops tea tree essential oil

6 cups distilled water

Steams are an amazing way to detoxify pores. They work effectively on their own, loosening debris, dirt and oil, but they are also great to use before a mask or other facial treatment because they allow the ingredients to thoroughly penetrate the skin. Doing at-home steams always makes me feel like I've been transported to a spa. This recipe makes 1 treatment, but you can do a double or triple batch and store it in the fridge for 1 week or so.

Combine herbs and tea tree oil in a glass jar and close tightly. Leave it overnight to "marinate."

To steam, add herbs and water to a large saucepan and bring to a boil. Once water has boiled, lower heat to a simmer. With thoroughly cleaned skin, lean your head over the saucepan, keeping your face about 1 foot away, with a towel over your head and the pot. Allow the steam to penetrate your skin for 15 minutes. Follow with a mask or moisturizer.

Pampering Recipes

Pampering skincare recipes are intended to help maintain beautiful skin or to just give yourself a special treat. We all deserve to indulge in a little pampering once a week . . . or once a day! A lot of these recipes make great gifts, it's essential to share the pampering love!

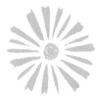

Hibiscus Glow Blush

$\frac{1}{2}$ teaspoon arrowroot powder or cornstarch
$\frac{1}{4}$ teaspoon hibiscus powder
Sprinkle of cocoa powder

Not only is formulating your own blush a great way to avoid harmful toxins and preservatives, but this recipe gives you the most natural, beautiful glow! Blend some up for yourself and for your friends.

Stir ingredients until they are thoroughly blended and one uniform color. Add more hibiscus powder or cocoa powder depending on the level of pink or warmth you want. Store in a small sifter jar and apply with a fluffy blush at the apples of the cheeks.

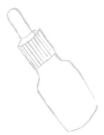

Aura Glow Highlighter

ALL

2 tablespoons grapeseed oil
1 teaspoon vitamin E oil
$\frac{1}{2}$ teaspoon zinc oxide powder
$1\frac{1}{2}$ teaspoons silver mica powder

Cosmetic highlighters are a beautiful way to give a glow to your skin. Not all of the ingredients for this recipe are available at the supermarket (though you can find them in online specialty stores), but the end result is worth the hunt and makes an extremely impressive gift!

Combine all ingredients in a small glass bottle and shake to combine. To use, apply to the tops of the cheekbones and inner corners of the eye for a hint of light, or blend a small amount with liquid foundation for an all-over glow.

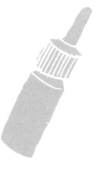

De-Puffing Cucumber-Aloe Eye Gel

½ cucumber, peeled and diced
¼ cup aloe vera gel
5 drops vitamin E oil

Puffy eyes are the worst; they give away the fact that you're lacking sleep, suffering from allergies or perhaps had a few too many the night before . . . not to mention they can be a bit painful! Cucumber and aloe de-puff and thoroughly soothe the eye area. You may forget how you got your puffy eyes to begin with!

Combine ingredients in blender, and blend until smooth. Pour into a small glass jar, seal and refrigerate for at least 2 hours. Pat onto clean, dry skin, focusing on the corners of the eyes.

Gel should last up to 3 weeks.

Dark Circle-Lightening Peach Treatment

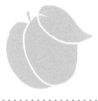

½ medium ripe peach
1 teaspoon aloe vera gel

Under-eye circles tend to make you look more tired than you actually are and can be pretty difficult to treat and conceal. Luckily, the high levels of vitamins A and E in peaches are amazing for combating darkness. This eye treatment is surprisingly effective and is beyond refreshing to tired, puffy eyes.

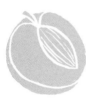

Dice the peach, including the skin, and then mash it into a paste using the back of a spoon, a fork or the blunt end of a knife. Stir in the aloe vera gel and combine thoroughly. Spread the mixture underneath your eyes and even on your lids if you like . . . just be careful not to get it in your eyes! Let sit for 20 minutes, and rinse thoroughly.

This treatment is incredibly gentle and can be done several times a week.

Beet Lip Stain

2 small beets, raw, peeled
4 drops fresh-squeezed lemon juice
¼ teaspoon unrefined virgin coconut oil

Beets are superfoods packed with vitamins, minerals and antioxidants, and anyone who's ever had any mishaps with them in the kitchen knows they can stain your skin for days at a time. Why not put that staining power to good use and use that beautiful beet-red hue as a lip stain?

For this recipe you'll want to wear gloves and lay down butcher paper to protect your hands and surfaces. Wash and cut beets and send them through a juicer into a small glass bowl. Add lemon juice and oil, and stir thoroughly. Transfer stain into a very small container using a dropper or a small funnel. Apply with a lip brush, or, even better, package your stain in a small rollerball container!

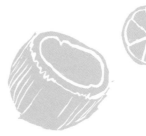

Cooling Mint Face Spray

2 bags mint tea
1 cup water
Juice of 1 lemon, strained
1 teaspoon vegetable glycerine
10 drops tea tree essential oil
10 drops peppermint essential oil

Whether it's a hot day, you're feeling flustered or your skin is inflamed and irritated, nothing feels better than cooling it down with a mint-infused spray. Keep this recipe in a spray bottle in the fridge, and spritz it on whenever you need to cool down!

Bring water to a boil in a medium saucepan, and remove from heat. Add tea bags and let steep for 8 to 10 minutes. Remove bags and let cool. Once tea has cooled, add juice, glycerine, tea tree oil and peppermint oil. Stir thoroughly, and transfer to spray bottle using a small funnel. Shake before use.

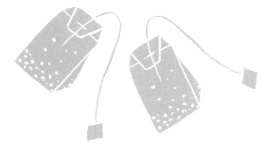

Strawberry Teeth Whitener

①   1 large strawberry or 2 small strawberries,
de-stemmed
½ teaspoon baking soda

This sounds incredibly vain, but for a very long time I was hesitant to switch over to natural dental products because I was worried I would have to compromise my pearly whites, thinking that nature couldn't give me the white teeth I desired. I couldn't have been more wrong. This tooth whitener is every bit as effective as store-bought strips and gels but is 100 percent safe and does not cause any sensitivity whatsoever. Baking soda penetrates deep stains, and the malic acid of strawberries whitens and brightens. You can't lose!

In a small bowl, mash strawberry using a fork. Sprinkle in baking soda, and continue to mash until a paste is formed. Spread mixture on your teeth and let sit for 5 to 10 minutes. Rinse, and brush teeth as usual.

Lemon-Sugar Face Scrub

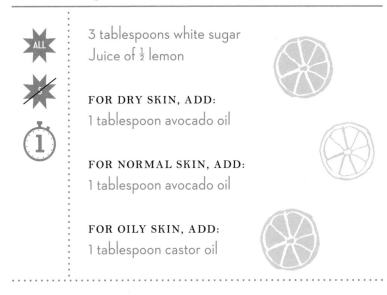

3 tablespoons white sugar

Juice of ½ lemon

FOR DRY SKIN, ADD:

1 tablespoon avocado oil

FOR NORMAL SKIN, ADD:

1 tablespoon avocado oil

FOR OILY SKIN, ADD:

1 tablespoon castor oil

This scrub is perfect for those dealing with some seriously dull skin. Sugar gently sloughs off dead skin, and lemon's vitamin C dissolves any left behind! Formulate this scrub with the oil intended for your skin type, and it will thoroughly nourish your skin as well.

Combine sugar with selected oil and stir until well blended. Stir in lemon juice. Gently massage scrub onto your skin, concentrating on areas of dullness or flakiness for 1 to 2 minutes. For optimal results, let the scrub sit on your skin for 5 minutes. Rinse or towel off.

Ingredient Spotlight
Lemon

emon is not just to add a bit of tartness to your iced tea: This little fruit packs a powerful beauty punch. Lemon is antibacterial and antifungal, therefore working wonders on acne-prone or congested skin. Chock-full of citric acid, lemons help to fade scars and lighten dark spots. Lemon on its own is so great, freshly squeezed juice can make a wonderful toner for oily or imbalanced skin.

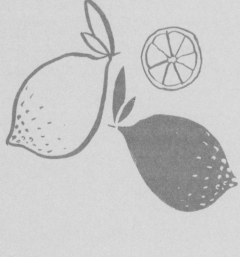

All-Natural Bronzing Powder

ALL

1 tablespoon cinnamon
1 teaspoon cocoa powder
1 teaspoon nutmeg
2 teaspoons cornstarch

My number one favorite makeup product is bronzer; it adds a beautiful, sun-kissed, healthy glow no matter what the season! Can you believe you can make an all-natural bronzer out of ingredients you probably already have in your kitchen? Take away the cornstarch, and it would also make a really yummy additive to your morning coffee—the beauty of Homemade Beauty!

Combine all ingredients and stir until the mixture is one uniform color. This recipe is definitely not strict, and you can play with the levels of cinnamon, cocoa powder and nutmeg until you achieve the perfect shade for your skin tone.

I love repurposing an empty mineral powder jar for storage of this bronzer because it allows me to use just the right amount. Brush a bit of your bronzer on your cheekbones, around your hairline and on your neck for a perfectly natural sun-kissed glow.

Coconut-Mango Lip Gloss

½ teaspoon unrefined virgin coconut oil
1 teaspoon fresh aloe vera gel
⅛ teaspoon vitamin E oil
3 drops natural mango extract

Supple, glossy lips without the toxins of regular cosmetics? Sign me up! This lip gloss is so delicious and adds an amazing sheen to your lips. Even better, it gives the added bonus of healing and soothing the lips.

Liquefy coconut oil by microwaving it for a few seconds or heating it on the stove in a small saucepan set over low heat.

Combine all ingredients in a small bowl and stir thoroughly. Pour into a resealable small jar or container before the mixture solidifies.

Apply gloss using your finger or a lip brush.

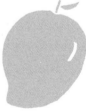

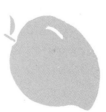

Mattifying Face Powder

2 tablespoons cornstarch or arrowroot powder
2 or more teaspoons of cocoa powder, depending
on the depth of your skin tone
5 drops lemon essential oil

Glowing skin is gorgeous; greasy skin on the other hand . . . let's just say that it's not the most flattering. This powder is fantastic for setting liquid foundation or for dusting on your T-zone throughout the day to keep oil at bay. Oh, and it's insanely easy to make!

Combine cornstarch and cocoa powder in a bowl, and then stir in the lemon essential oil until the powder is one uniform color. Apply a test on the side of your face to determine whether you need to add more cocoa powder, adding a ½ teaspoon at a time as necessary.

For ideal storage and application, transfer powder to a recycled mineral face-powder jar and dust on lightly with a fluffy brush on clean skin, to set liquid foundation or to touch up throughout the day.

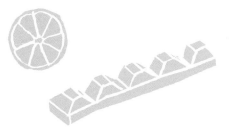

At-Home Microdermabrasion

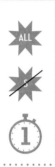

2 teaspoons baking soda
½ teaspoon distilled water
½ teaspoon freshly squeezed lemon juice
5 drops lavender essential oil

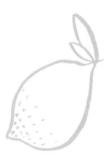

Microdermabrasion is an incredible tool for reducing scarring, dark spots and hyper pigmentation, but it certainly isn't cheap and isn't always the safest. This recipe is about as close as it gets to a spa microdermabrasion using all natural ingredients! Microdermabrasion may have a sensitizing effect on the skin, so this treatment is best done in the evening.

Combine the ingredients in a bowl, and use your fingers to thoroughly stir until a paste is formed. Gently massage the paste onto your skin in small, circular motions for 5 minutes. Remove with a moist hot towel, using soft, swiping motions, careful to not do any additional scrubbing. Pat face with cool water.

You may experience redness for a couple of hours, so make sure not to aggravate your skin with any more facial treatments or makeup application. Be sure to wear sunscreen the next time you are exposed to sun.

Lash-Growth Serum

1 tablespoon castor oil
1 tablespoon almond oil
5 drops vitamin E oil

Unfortunately, not all of us were born with the lashes that are achieved by applying mascara, false lashes or lash extensions, all of which can be costly, time-consuming and difficult to use and potentially damaging to your natural lashes. There are several pharmacological-grade lash-growth serums on the market, but they contain strong chemicals that may be harmful to your health. This all-natural lash-growth serum will plump and strengthen your lashes, encouraging their growth and retention.

Combine all ingredients in a small glass jar or bottle and shake thoroughly to combine. Always shake before use. At night, dip a clean mascara wand (packs of these can be purchased at any beauty-supply store) into your serum and brush through your lashes, concentrating your application at the roots. Try to avoid getting too much in your eyes (it won't hurt you, but the serum will feel strange and uncomfortable). Leave on overnight, and rinse in the morning. For optimal results, you can also apply a small amount to your lashes on days you won't be wearing any eye makeup.

Berry-Tinted Lip Balm

2 or 3 small berries (blackberries, strawberries or
    raspberries)
1 tablespoon beeswax
1 teaspoon unrefined virgin coconut oil

I am a self-proclaimed lip balm junkie . . . like many people, I can't get enough of the stuff. Even better is tinted lip balm—it has the ease of application of lip balm but with a beautiful rosy tint. It's a casual girl's best friend. Making your own berry-tinted lip balm is a lot of fun. Play around with different berries to find your perfect tint!

Over low heat, liquefy berries and then strain out any seeds or chunks. In a double boiler set over low heat, melt beeswax and coconut oil. Remove from heat and stir in berry juice. Pour into a resealable small tin or jar and allow to cool before placing the lid on.

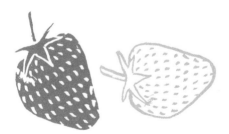

chapter 5

Hair

. . . .

Our hair craves natural, nutrient-dense, food-grade products as much as our bodies do. In this chapter you'll find recipes for shampoos, conditioners, masks, treatments and even styling products. You'll be amazed by how fast your hair responds to some of these treatments, by the difference in your hair's health over time and by how much money you'll save using hand-crafted products!

Cleansing Recipes

Whether your hair is dry, oily, or normal, you can make your own shampoo at home! There's even a recipe for an all-natural dry shampoo . . . once you try it, you'll never buy another chemical-filled version again!

The most important thing you need to know about natural shampoos is that they are far less stripping than the store-bought versions and much better at preserving your hair's natural and protective oils (trust me, you want those), but due to product buildup that a lot of us inevitably have from years of commercial styling products and conditioners, you may want to use a clarifying rinse (like my Olive Oil–Lemon Clarifying Shampoo, page 82) before trying these shampoos for the first time. It will make your transition to homemade shampoos a bit easier!

Invigorating Grapefruit-Mint Shampoo

N/O

¼ cup liquid castile soap
¼ cup distilled water
1 teaspoon vegetable glycerine
Juice of ½ grapefruit, strained
20 drops peppermint essential oil

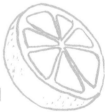

This recipe makes your hair feel squeaky-clean without over drying it, like store-bought shampoos with their harsh ingredients can. Grapefruit gently exfoliates the scalp, allowing peppermint oil to penetrate, stimulate and balance the scalp's pH levels.

Combine ingredients in a recycled shampoo bottle or resealable container of your choice. Shake thoroughly before each use. Apply a small amount to scalp, lather and massage for 1 to 2 minutes. Rinse thoroughly, and follow with conditioner.

Tea Tree-Jojoba Dandruff Shampoo

ALL

$\frac{1}{4}$ cup liquid castile soap

$\frac{1}{2}$ cup distilled water

1 teaspoon vegetable glycerine

2 tablespoons jojoba oil

20 drops tea tree essential oil

Tea tree oil is fabulous for ridding the scalp of dandruff, but it tends to be quite drying for some people and can further aggravate the condition. Jojoba oil is a lightweight oil that is easily absorbed by the skin, as it is so similar to our body's natural sebum. Combine the two together in a shampoo, and you have the perfect recipe for dandruff elimination and scalp hydration!

In a recycled shampoo bottle or squeeze bottle container, combine all ingredients. Shake before each use, applying a small amount to wet hair. Lather and massage shampoo into scalp thoroughly. For best results, let it sit on your scalp for at least 5 minutes. Rinse thoroughly, and follow with conditioner.

Ingredient Spotlight
Tea Tree Oil

A lot of people spend tons of time and money blasting their skin and scalp with chemicals in order to get relief from all sorts of inflammations and disorders. Tea tree oil is antifungal and antiseptic, making it especially effective in treating acne and dandruff. Make sure that you purchase only 100 percent pure tea tree oil.

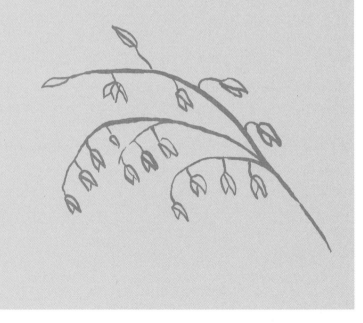

All-Natural Dry Shampoo

 ½ cup arrowroot powder or cornstarch
10 drops essential oil of your choice

Dry shampoo, which is used to absorb excess oil on the scalp or add texture and body to hair, is an incredibly useful product. Unfortunately, using it frequently (which most dry shampoo lovers do) can get pretty pricey. You will not believe how easy, inexpensive and effective this DIY dry shampoo is.

In a small bowl, combine ingredients and stir together until the oil has completely dissipated. Use a funnel to transfer dry shampoo to a recycled old salt shaker. To use, sprinkle onto scalp and thoroughly scrub in using "shampooing" motions.

If you're a brunette and have problems getting the dry shampoo to blend in with your scalp, try adjusting the powder levels to ¼ cup arrowroot powder or cornstarch and ¼ cup cocoa powder.

Highlight-Enhancing Chamomile Shampoo

1 cup distilled water
6 bags chamomile tea
½ cup liquid castile soap
1 tablespoon vegetable glycerine
Juice of ½ lemon

Chamomile flowers make a delicious, soothing tea, but they also have the ability to subtly lighten your hair. Due to chamomile's calming capabilities, this shampoo is also great if you have a dry, irritated scalp!

Bring water to a boil in a medium saucepan set over high heat. Remove from heat, add tea bags and let steep in the saucepan for 30 minutes. Discard tea bags and let mixture cool. Combine tea with remaining ingredients in a recycled shampoo bottle or any other flip-top bottle.

To use, shake thoroughly and apply a small amount to wet hair. Lather and massage into scalp, then rinse thoroughly. Follow with conditioner.

Depth-Enhancing Black Tea Shampoo

N/D

1 cup distilled water
6 bags unsweetened, unflavored black tea
½ cup liquid castile soap
1 tablespoon vegetable glycerine
10 drops ylang ylang essential oil

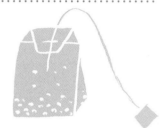

Dark hair is so mysterious and gorgeous, but with our environment, certain shampoos and water types can often dull rich brunette tones. With repeated use, this black tea shampoo will enhance your dark hair and give it a lustrous shine.

Bring water to a boil in a medium saucepan. Remove from heat, add tea bags and steep for 30 minutes. Remove tea bags and allow tea to cool completely. Combine tea with remaining ingredients and transfer to resealable container of your choice. To use, squirt a small amount into hands and work into a lather. Apply to scalp and massage. Let the shampoo sit for 2 minutes, then rinse thoroughly. Follow with conditioner.

Coconut-Lavender Shampoo

1 teaspoon unrefined virgin coconut oil
$\frac{2}{3}$ cup liquid castile soap
$\frac{1}{2}$ cup coconut milk
$\frac{1}{4}$ cup distilled water
1 teaspoon vitamin E oil
5 drops lavender essential oil

So many shampoos are filled with harsh cleansing agents, which can dehydrate and strip your locks; this super gentle yet thoroughly cleansing shampoo is kind to your coif and makes your hair smell incredible. I love this shampoo because it's super easy to whip up!

Melt coconut oil in the microwave for 15 to 30 seconds or in a double boiler. Combine all of the ingredients in an empty squeeze bottle and shake until thoroughly blended. Shake before each use. Shampoo as normal, follow with conditioner and enjoy your beautifully scented hair!

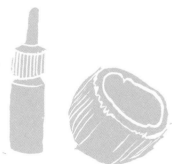

Avocado-Aloe Shampoo

N/D

½ cup distilled water
¼ cup liquid castile soap
¼ cup aloe vera gel
1 tablespoon avocado oil
1 tablespoon vegetable glycerine

This recipe makes a wonderful hydrating, gentle shampoo that I especially love to use if my scalp has gotten sunburned. Avocado hydrates and nourishes while aloe deeply soothes.

Combine ingredients in a blender and blend on low or mix with a hand mixer until the aloe vera gel has been mixed in thoroughly. Transfer to shampoo container and shake gently to combine. To use, shake gently, work a small amount into a lather between your palms and apply to wet hair, concentrating on the scalp. Rinse thoroughly, and follow with conditioner.

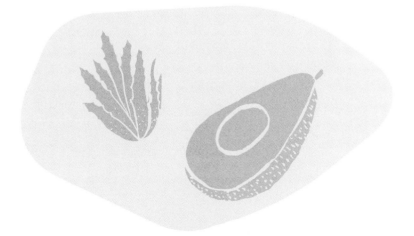

Olive Oil–Lemon Clarifying Shampoo

N/O

½ cup distilled water

½ cup liquid castile soap

1 tablespoon glycerine

Juice of 1 lemon

2 teaspoons extra-virgin olive oil

10 drops lemon essential oil

Sweat, poor water quality, product buildup and flaky scalp are all reasons to clarify your hair. It's important to cleanse the hair of residue, but you don't want to strip it entirely of its natural protective oils. The lemon in this recipe gently cleanses the scalp and hair of debris, and olive oil ensures hydration and nourishment.

Combine all ingredients into a plastic squeeze bottle, and shake gently until combined. To use, start by rinsing hair thoroughly; let the water of your shower do as much work as it can to remove existing product residue. Work a generous amount of this shampoo between your hands to create a lather and massage into scalp, letting it penetrate down the length of your hair. Rinse thoroughly, and follow with conditioner.

Moisturizing Recipes

Just like moisture is essential to the skin, it is also imperative for hair. It's so important to keep the hair hydrated . . . not only will this protect it from outside elements, but it will keep it looking and feeling its healthiest.

This section contains recipes for everyday conditioner to intensive hydrating treatments.

Coconut-Lavender Conditioner

N/D

1½ teaspoons guar gum

1 teaspoon unrefined virgin coconut oil

1 cup coconut milk

15 drops lavender essential oil

In my opinion, there's not much more soothing and luxurious than the scent of lavender. Combine that with hydrating coconut, and you have a super-indulgent conditioner that is still light enough to use every day!

Combine all ingredients in a squeeze bottle, and shake vigorously until ingredients are thoroughly combined and there are no clumps. To use, apply generously after shampooing. Rinse thoroughly.

Shea Butter Hair Treatment

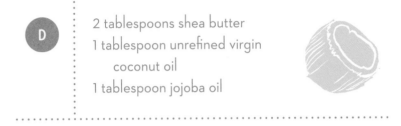

D

2 tablespoons shea butter
1 tablespoon unrefined virgin
    coconut oil
1 tablespoon jojoba oil

Relieving frizzy, brittle hair, this treatment is for the driest of manes. You'll see a dramatic difference in your hair after just one use, but when used regularly once a week, after a couple of months you'll have what feels like brand-new hair!

Melt shea butter and coconut oil in a double boiler until liquefied. Remove from heat, and stir in jojoba oil. Let cool in the fridge until solidified. After solidification, whip with a hand mixer until a creamy consistency has been reached.

To use, apply to freshly shampooed hair, and let sit for at least 20 minutes and up to overnight. Rinse thoroughly, and style as usual.

Honey Hair Smoothie

ALL

①

2 tablespoons honey
1 cup plain yogurt
1 teaspoon unrefined virgin coconut oil

Hydration is important, but too much of a good thing can weigh down hair and make it look stringy and oily. This hair smoothie gives your hair the hydration it needs and locks in moisture long term while ensuring that your hair maintains bounce and body.

Place ingredients in a blender, and blend on low until combined. To use, apply mixture to dry hair, and let sit for 15 minutes. Rinse thoroughly, shampoo and follow with conditioner.

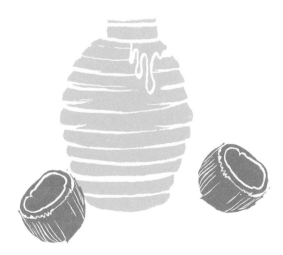

Hydrating Rose Water Hair Mist

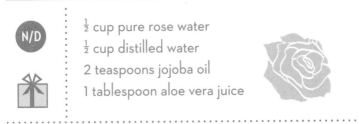

½ cup pure rose water

½ cup distilled water

2 teaspoons jojoba oil

1 tablespoon aloe vera juice

Rose water is one of the loveliest all-natural beautifiers. It smells incredible, lightly hydrates and gives a beautiful glow . . . not only to your skin but to your hair, too! This mist works as a style prep or as a pick-me-up for curly or wavy hair.

Combine all ingredients in a spritz bottle and shake thoroughly to combine. Spritz on damp hair before styling or onto dry curls or waves that need a lift.

Banana-Honey Dry Scalp Treatment

ALL

½ banana
2 tablespoons honey

①

Banana and honey are both extremely hydrating without being oily or greasy. This recipe is perfect for anyone with a tight, dry, flaky scalp or someone wanting to improve the condition of their hair; healthy hair starts with a healthy scalp!

Mash banana thoroughly, and stir in honey until mixture is smooth. Wet hair for optimal absorption and apply treatment to scalp, working through to the ends of your hair if desired (this mask is just as good for your hair as it is for your scalp!). Let treatment sit for at least 30 minutes, then rinse. Follow with shampoo and conditioner.

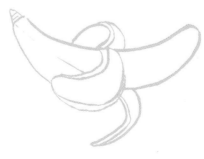

Ingredient Spotlight
Honey

You'll see honey mentioned a number of times in the recipes of this book, and that's because it is an extremely valuable topical beauty product. Honey cleanses; moisturizes; contains tons of minerals like iron, phosphorous and magnesium; and also acts as an anti-inflammatory. Just make sure you are using high-quality, raw, unprocessed honey in your *Homemade Beauty* concoctions!

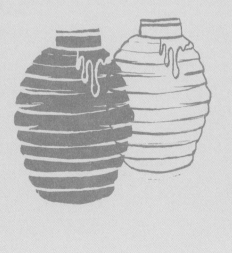

Avocado-Honey Revitalizing Hair Treatment

D

1

½ avocado, cubed
1 tablespoon honey
½ tablespoon unrefined virgin coconut oil
½ tablespoon extra-virgin olive oil

Whenever my hair is feeling brittle, dull and extremely dry, I turn to this recipe. This heavy-hitting concoction targets all the woes of dry hair. Avocado nourishes and strengthens, honey rids the scalp of unwanted bacteria while acting as a humectant, coconut oil deeply hydrates and olive oil adds beautiful shine. If you want to use this recipe but have oily hair, simply reduce the amount of oil in the recipe or leave it out altogether.

Thoroughly mash avocado; then stir in the remaining ingredients until smooth and blended. Apply treatment all over hair and scalp, making sure to thoroughly coat ends. For best results, cover hair with plastic wrap. Let sit for 30 minutes, and rinse thoroughly. Follow with shampoo and conditioner.

Invigorating Coffee Conditioning Rinse

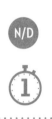

N/D

1 cup coffee, cooled
1 cup coconut milk
1 teaspoon jojoba oil

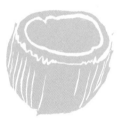

This coffee conditioner invigorates the scalp, gives your hair incredible shine and hydrates as well. If you're a coffee lover, this is definitely the conditioner for you!

Combine ingredients in a squeeze or flip-top bottle and shake to combine. Pour through shampooed, wet hair, and let sit for at least 2 minutes. Rinse thoroughly, and style as usual.

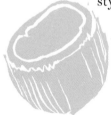

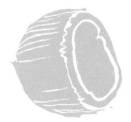

After-Sun Hydrating Hair Treatment

ALL

1

¼ cup fresh aloe vera gel
1 tablespoon sweet almond oil
¼ cup coconut milk
20 drops lavender essential oil

Just like you'd care for your skin if you spent too much time in the sun, it's important to take care of your hair if it's undergone excessive sun exposure; UV rays can be very damaging to hair. Even if intense sun on your scalp doesn't feel as painful as a sunburn on your skin does, sun exposure can be a big shock to your strands. This recipe replenishes the hair and soothes the scalp, keeping your hair strong and healthy.

Blend, mix or thoroughly stir ingredients together until smooth. After shampooing, apply treatment to scalp and hair and let it sit for 20 minutes. Rinse thoroughly, and follow with conditioner.

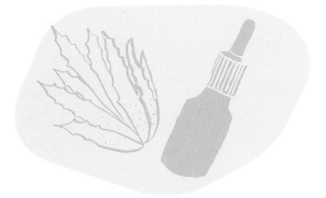

Strengthening Banana Hair Mask

N/D

1

$\frac{1}{2}$ banana

1 egg

1 tablespoon unrefined virgin coconut oil

$\frac{1}{2}$ tablespoon honey

Bananas are some serious multitaskers not only when it comes to health (gotta love that potassium) but in the beauty department, too. Banana contains pantothenic acid, which strengthens the hair. The wonderfully humectant honey draws moisture to the hair, and the egg's protein reinforces your follicles. This mask is great for those of you wanting to grow your hair and prevent it from breaking!

Mash the banana until smooth. In a separate bowl, beat the egg until frothy. Combine all of the ingredients in a small bowl and stir until thoroughly blended. Shampoo, and then apply to scalp and hair. Leave on for no longer than 20 minutes (egg tends to be drying to the hair if left on too long). Rinse thoroughly, and condition.

Ingredient Spotlight
Banana

Bananas should be included in everyone's diets for their numerous health benefits, but we could all also profit from slathering some banana on our skin and hair. Full of B vitamins, banana nourishes the skin and hair while fighting dryness and flakiness. It is also great at balancing skin, making it perfect for combination skin.

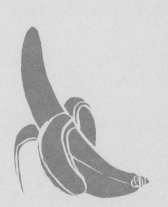

Protein-Enriching Hair Treatment

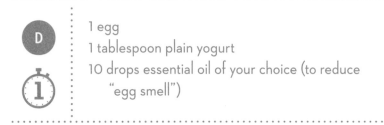

1 egg
1 tablespoon plain yogurt
10 drops essential oil of your choice (to reduce "egg smell")

Our hair is mostly protein, and when it is not supported and nourished, hair can feel dry and brittle and break easily. Eggs and yogurt are incredible sources of protein, not only for our bodies but for our hair, too.

In a small bowl, beat together egg, yogurt and essential oil. After shampooing, apply treatment generously to hair, concentrating on your scalp. Leave on for 20 minutes, rinse thoroughly and follow with conditioner.

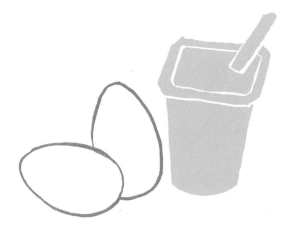

Split End–Banishing Treatment

1 teaspoon extra-virgin olive oil
1 teaspoon unrefined virgin coconut oil
1 teaspoon sweet olive oil
$\frac{1}{2}$ teaspoon honey

Split ends are such a pesky annoyance, but they are a warning sign from our bodies that hair isn't receiving enough nourishment. Make sure to use a scalp treatment for your specific needs, and use this recipe to fortify and strengthen your ends.

Place ingredients in a small saucepan over low heat and stir until melted and thoroughly combined. Remove from heat and apply to dry hair, from mid-shaft to the ends. Leave on for at least 30 minutes, but this treatment can be left on as long as overnight (just be sure to sleep with a shower cap on in order to avoid getting the oils on your skin and pillow).

Rinse thoroughly, shampoo and condition.

You can also make a modification of this recipe without honey, and apply a very small amount to ends after styling.

Conditioning Styling Hair Pomade

⅛ cup beeswax

¼ cup shea butter

1 teaspoon unrefined virgin coconut oil

2 tablespoons jojoba oil

2 tablespoons arrowroot powder

10 drops essential oil of your choice

Pomade is great for defining and holding the hair as well as taming flyaways. I love this recipe because not only does it accomplish the aforementioned, it conditions hair at the same time.

Melt beeswax and shea butter in a double boiler set over low to medium heat. Stir in coconut oil and remove from heat. In a separate small bowl, combine jojoba oil with arrowroot powder. Combine the arrowroot paste with the beeswax, shea butter and coconut oil, and stir in essential oil. Transfer pomade to a blender and blend on low speed until smooth. Pour into a resealable tin or small jar and let cool overnight.

To use, work a small amount of product between your palms and use to style short hair, smooth down flyaways, work midshaft down to add texture or apply to ends to disguise split ends and dryness.

Honey-Banana Shine Mask

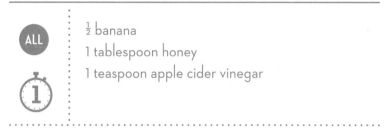

ALL

(1)

½ banana
1 tablespoon honey
1 teaspoon apple cider vinegar

We've already established that honey and banana make great hair hydrators, which can definitely help hair shine, but residue-reducing apple cider vinegar can take your shine to the next level!

Mash banana until completely smooth, and stir in honey and apple cider vinegar. Ensure that your ingredients are totally blended to allow for proper distribution. Apply mixture to shampooed hair, and let sit for 15 minutes. Rinse thoroughly, and follow with conditioner.

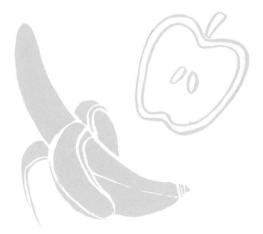

Coconut Shine Serum

2 tablespoons unrefined virgin coconut oil
1 tablespoon castor oil
½ teaspoon vitamin E oil
10 drops rose essential oil

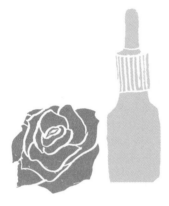

I'm addicted to shine serums; I love how healthy they make my hair look. Unfortunately, most serums on the market are mostly comprised of silicone, which coats the hair with plasticizers and gives only a temporary appearance of healthy hair, in addition to suffocating the scalp and causing unwanted buildup. This recipe not only gives you the shine you want but improves the health of your hair.

If solidified, melt coconut oil in a small saucepan over low heat. Stir coconut oil, castor oil, vitamin E oil and essential oil together, and transfer to a resealable small bottle or container.

To use, rub a couple of drops between your palms and rake through damp hair. You can also press it onto dried, styled hair for added shine and to reduce flyaways.

Frizz-Taming Hair Serum

N/D

2 tablespoons castor oil
1 tablespoon avocado oil
½ tablespoon extra-virgin olive oil
10 drops essential oil of your choice

Frizzy hair can be terribly frustrating—it's difficult to manage and not always the most attractive of looks. This serum tames frizz and conditions the hair without weighing it down.

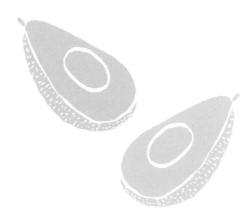

Combine ingredients in a resealable small bottle or container. To use, shake container to blend. Pour a couple of drops onto your palm, rub together and then pat onto dry hair.

Avocado-Coconut Reparative Hair Mask

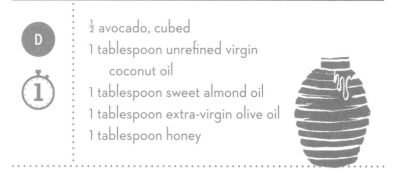

D

①

½ avocado, cubed
1 tablespoon unrefined virgin
    coconut oil
1 tablespoon sweet almond oil
1 tablespoon extra-virgin olive oil
1 tablespoon honey

Even occasional heat styling, coloring and UV or chlorine exposure can leave your locks crying out for help. This reparative mask works wonders for strengthening and hydrating your hair, while giving it a whole lot of shine. (Side note: This was the first Homemade Beauty product I whipped up at home!)

Mash the avocado up in a bowl until smooth, and then add the remaining ingredients. Stir until mixture is thoroughly blended.

Apply to dry hair, and let concoction sit for 20 minutes and up to 1 hour. Rinse thoroughly, and shampoo, condition and style as usual.

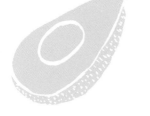

De-Frizzing Hair Rinse

N/D

3 cups distilled water
1 tablespoon raw honey
1 teaspoon jojoba oil

Honey acts as a humectant, which draws moisture into skin and hair. Properly hydrated hair is de-frizzed hair. This rinse cuts frizz without weighing down your hair!

Warm water in a medium saucepan set over low to medium heat, and stir in honey and jojoba oil until honey has dissolved. Remove from heat, allow to cool and transfer to a squeeze bottle.

Pour through hair after shampooing, and let sit for 5 minutes before rinsing. Follow with conditioner, if desired.

Detoxifying Recipes

Styling products, conditioners and the environment can create buildup, causing hair to look dull and unhealthy. Most of us are focused on constantly hydrating the hair, but detoxifying and reducing buildup is just as important—if there is too much buildup on the hair, conditioning ingredients have no way of reaching your hair and scalp! Find the recipes that work for you, and use them twice a month!

Brown Sugar Exfoliating Scalp Treatment

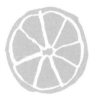

D

1

1 tablespoon brown sugar
½ tablespoon jojoba oil
½ tablespoon extra-virgin
   olive oil
Juice of ½ lemon

Scalp buildup can cause dullness and flakes. You want to ensure that your scalp is clear, without making it dry and tight. This treatment removes buildup and flakes but is infused with hydrating oils.

Stir ingredients together in a small bowl until thoroughly blended. When hair is dry, apply treatment generously to scalp and gently massage for 1 to 2 minutes. Let sit for 10 minutes. Rinse thoroughly, and follow with shampoo and conditioner.

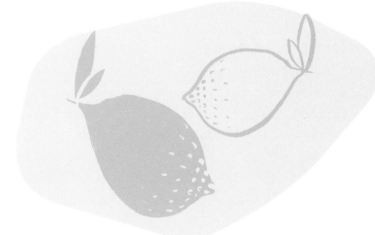

Detoxifying Carrot Hair Treatment

N/O

(1)

1 large carrot, boiled and
   mashed
1 tablespoon yogurt
1 teaspoon honey
Juice of ½ lemon

Carrots have tons of vitamins and keep your eyes strong, but they also work wonders to revitalize and cleanse the hair. This treatment is ideal for when your hair is looking limp and dull due to product buildup or excessive oil.

Stir ingredients together or combine in a food processor or blender until smooth. Generously apply to dry hair, and let sit for up to 30 minutes. Rinse thoroughly, and follow with shampoo and conditioner.

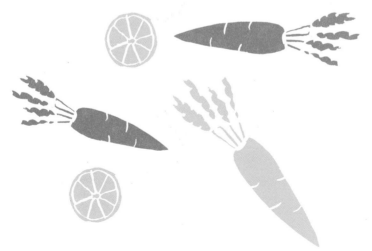

Lemon-Aloe Oil-Reducing Rinse

N/O

①

Juice of ½ lemon
1 tablespoon aloe vera gel
1 teaspoon apple cider vinegar
1 cup distilled water

Some of us produce a great amount of oil from our scalps, which is great for scalp and hair health but can make hair look limp, stringy or lifeless. This rinse helps reduce oil on the scalp and hair without stripping it of essential nutrients.

Whisk ingredients together or combine in a food processor. Transfer to a squeeze bottle or spouted container, pour through shampooed hair and let sit for 5 minutes. Rinse thoroughly, and follow with conditioner.

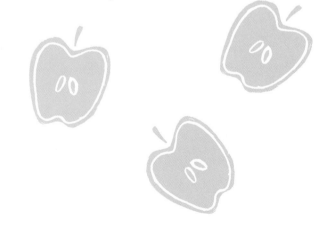

Clarifying Baking Soda Rinse

1 tablespoon baking soda
1 cup distilled water

Did you go overboard with your deep conditioner? Are you a little heavy-handed with hair oils and serums? Product buildup can completely negate the intended effects of styling products. This rinse

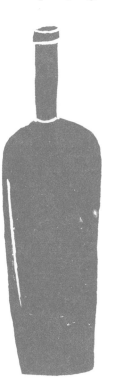

wipes out buildup in minutes and leaves your hair ready to receive moisture again . . . just take it easy with the application! Use this treatment sparingly, as extended use can over-dry your hair.

Combine ingredients in a spray or squeeze bottle. Shake thoroughly, distribute throughout dry hair and let sit for 1 to 2 minutes. Rinse thoroughly, and follow with shampoo and conditioner.

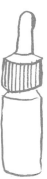

Tea Tree Invigorating Scalp Spray

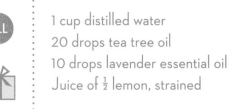

1 cup distilled water
20 drops tea tree oil
10 drops lavender essential oil
Juice of ½ lemon, strained

What if your scalp feels itchy, tight, flaky or just flat-out gross and you don't have the time to do a full-on treatment or mask? This invigorating, refreshing and detoxifying scalp pick-me-up in a bottle is your answer.

Combine ingredients in a spray bottle. Shake thoroughly, and spritz sparingly onto dry scalp.

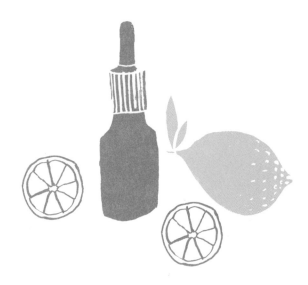

Restorative Rosemary-Citrus Treatment

1 cup distilled water
2 tablespoons dried rosemary
Juice of $\frac{1}{4}$ lemon
Juice of $\frac{1}{4}$ orange
1 teaspoon jojoba oil

Rosemary is probably the last thing you would think to use for beautifying, but it actually does a fantastic job of stimulating and clarifying the scalp, accounting for healthy hair growth. Combine it with nourishing and exfoliating citrus fruits and restorative jojoba oil, and you have a clarifying, detoxifying and strengthening treatment.

Bring water to a boil in a small saucepan, and add the dried rosemary. Remove the pan from heat and let the rosemary steep for at least 1 hour and up to overnight. Strain the herbs, and combine water with the remaining ingredients. Transfer treatment to a squeeze bottle. Shake bottle until ingredients are combined and pour over shampooed hair. Let sit for 10 minutes, rinse thoroughly and follow with conditioner.

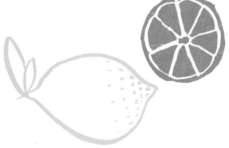

Apple Cider Vinegar and Lemon Hair Rinse

1 cup distilled water
2 tablespoons apple cider vinegar
Juice of ½ lemon

As much as I'm all about moisturizing my hair, every once in a while it's important to do a clarifying rinse to remove any residue. The best part about this rinse is that while it removes dulling product, buildup and dandruff, it also imparts a healthy shine.

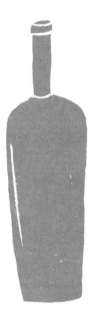

Combine all ingredients in a squeeze bottle or spouted cup for easy application. After shampooing, evenly pour the rinse over your scalp and through your hair. Give your scalp a nice massage, and rinse thoroughly with cool water. Follow with conditioner to remove any unwanted vinegar smell.

Apple Cider Vinegar

Apple cider vinegar may smell more like a salad dressing than a beauty tool, but don't let its pungent scent cause you to overlook its fantastic capabilities. Apple cider vinegar is wonderful for balancing the pH of the face and scalp, which soothes and gives you a more even tone. It also helps eliminate dead skin cells and buildup on the hair!

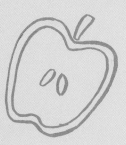

Coconut-Tea Tree Miracle Scalp Treatment

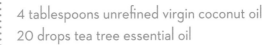

ALL

4 tablespoons unrefined virgin coconut oil
20 drops tea tree essential oil

I call this the "miracle scalp treatment" because it has truly worked magic on my scalp! The other miraculous aspect of it is that it's only two easy ingredients. The moment I notice any flaking on my scalp, I pop the treatment on and my crown is in the clear for weeks! This recipe makes just 1 treatment, but you can mix up a big batch and store it in a cool, dry place.

If solidified, melt coconut oil for 15 seconds in the microwave or in a small saucepan set over low heat. Stir the coconut oil and tea tree oil together until thoroughly blended. On dry hair, apply mixture into your scalp and massage for 1 to 2 minutes. Let sit for at least 2 hours, or you can even put your hair in a plastic shower cap or wrap it in plastic wrap and leave it overnight.

To remove, rinse thoroughly, shampoo (you may have to up to three times in order to get all of the oil out of your hair) and condition with a lightweight conditioner.

Cucumber–Olive Oil After-Pool Hair Revitalizer

ALL

½ cucumber, peeled and chopped
1 tablespoon extra-virgin olive oil
2 tablespoons distilled water

The chlorine and chemicals in pools can strip and drastically dry your hair, so it's important to take special care after taking a dip. Cucumbers are 95 percent water, making them great for replenishing hair hydration in a snap. Use this treatment, which cleanses the hair of chlorine while rehydrating it, after each time you swim, or twice a week if you're an everyday swimmer.

Blend ingredients in a food processor or blender on low to medium speed until smooth. Apply to hair right after the pool, and let sit for at least 10 minutes. Rinse, and follow with shampoo and conditioner.

If you're swimming on the go, you can keep this revitalizer in a spray bottle in your pool bag and spritz on after getting out of the water! Just rinse, shampoo and condition when you get home!

Pampering Recipes

From the environment to product buildup to heat styling, your hair takes a beating on a daily basis. It's important to treat your hair well and be sure to pamper it from time to time . . . and when you do style it, use gentle, mild styling products!

In this section there are recipes for all sorts of styling products, serums and even a hair perfume!

All-Natural Hair Spray

ALL

1 cup distilled water
2 tablespoons white sugar
1 tablespoon high-proof vodka
10 drops essential oil of your choice

Obviously we all want our perfectly coiffed hair to stay in place all day, but most hair sprays contain harmful chemicals and can dry and damage hair. This recipe, on the other hand, is all-natural and gentle to hair. The only problem? You have to be twenty-one or older to get all of the proper ingredients!

Bring water to a boil, and stir in sugar until it has dissolved. Remove from heat, and allow to cool. Stir in remaining ingredients, transfer to a spray bottle and use anytime you need to give your hair some hold!

Hair-Lightening Citrus Mist

ALL

2 cups distilled water
Juice of 2 lemons, strained
2 teaspoons unrefined virgin
    coconut oil
20 drops chamomile essential oil

Sun-kissed strands look beautiful in the summer, but sometimes the sun's effects are a bit more subtle than we'd like. This mist helps enhance the sun's hair-lightening effect and also refreshes and cools! If you're looking to lighten your hair, this is the perfect product to keep in your pool or beach bag or to carry along with you while camping, hiking or just spending the day outdoors.

Combine ingredients in a spray bottle. Shake thoroughly, and spritz over your hair before sun exposure. Repeat application every 2 hours.

Sun-Protection Serum

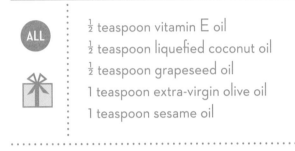

$\frac{1}{2}$ teaspoon vitamin E oil

$\frac{1}{2}$ teaspoon liquefied coconut oil

$\frac{1}{2}$ teaspoon grapeseed oil

1 teaspoon extra-virgin olive oil

1 teaspoon sesame oil

We love the sun for how it helps nourish the earth and our bodies, but too much sun isn't a good thing. Overexposure to the sun is pretty easy to achieve, but luckily this serum helps keep your hair (the first point of contact for the sun) nourished and protected.

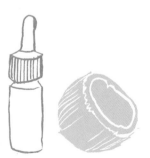

Combine ingredients in a small squeeze bottle. To use, shake bottle until ingredients are thoroughly blended, and rub a couple of drops between palms. Press over dry hair before and after sun exposure.

Coconut–Sea Salt Beach Waves Spray

½ cup coconut milk
½ cup distilled water
1 tablespoon sea salt
1 teaspoon unrefined virgin
   coconut oil

My all-time favorite hair style is tousled, beachy waves. Despite the fact it's a super-summery style, I tend to rock them year 'round. I've tried every store-bought beach wave spray on the market, and they leave my hair stiff, dry or stringy. This all-natural recipe gives you perfect, hydrated beach waves.

In a small saucepan, warm coconut milk and water over low heat. Stir in sea salt and coconut oil until fully dissolved. Allow to cool, and transfer to a spray bottle. To use, spray on damp hair and allow to air-dry.

If you'd like your wave spray to also double as a hair lightener, just add the juice of 1 lemon.

Black Tea Rinse for Deepening Brunette Hair

① 2 cups water
1 tablespoon jojoba oil
6 bags black tea

As a brunette, there's nothing I love more than having dark, glossy locks, but oftentimes the elements can leave my hair looking dull and rusty. This rinse naturally deepens brunette hair, while adding shine . . . plus it has the added benefit of enhancing hair growth!

Bring water to a boil, and then remove from heat. Stir in jojoba oil, add tea bags and let steep for at least 1 hour. Transfer to a squeeze bottle or spouted container. After shampooing, pour rinse all over hair and scalp. Let sit for 30 minutes, wrapping hair with plastic wrap or a plastic shower cap for best results. Rinse thoroughly, and follow with conditioner.

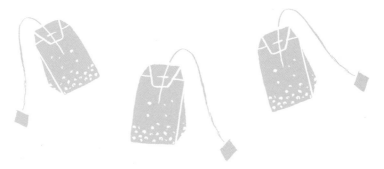

Lemon-Chamomile Lightening Rinse

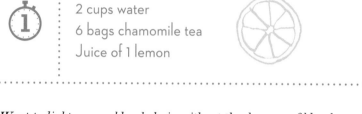

2 cups water
6 bags chamomile tea
Juice of 1 lemon

Want to lighten your blonde hair without the damage of bleach or peroxide? This rinse lightens and brightens your hair while soothing your scalp.

In a medium saucepan, bring water to a boil. Remove from heat, add tea bags and steep for at least 1 hour. Remove and discard tea bags, stir in lemon juice and transfer mixture to a squeeze bottle or spouted cup. On shampooed and rinsed hair, pour rinse through, and let sit for 10 minutes. Rinse thoroughly, and follow with conditioner.

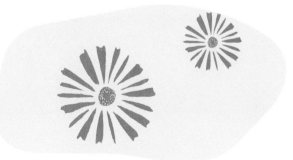

Damage-Healing Shine Serum

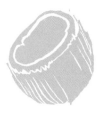

D

½ teaspoon unrefined virgin coconut oil
1 teaspoon jojoba oil
1 teaspoon grapeseed oil

In my opinion, there's nothing better than a product that makes your hair look incredible while deeply repairing damage and dryness— otherwise, what's the point of using it at all? This serum works to repair the structure of the hair shaft and provides essential hydration and nutrition.

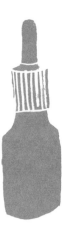

If coconut oil is solidified, place in a small dish in the microwave for 10 seconds to soften or melt. Stir in the remaining oils, and transfer to a small bottle. To use, rub a couple of drops between your palms and work through damp or dry hair.

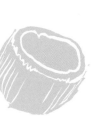

Hair Perfume

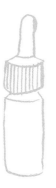

½ tablespoon jojoba oil
1 tablespoon fresh aloe vera gel
2 tablespoons distilled water
20 drops essential oil of your preference

I love clean-smelling hair, but for some, shampooing every day can be extremely stripping and drying and is just not an option. This hair perfume is perfect for when you want to freshen up without having to wet your hair, or serves as an excellent pick-me-up throughout a long day! Crafting hair perfume is a lot of fun, and even more so when you gather a group of friends and make it together!

Stir oil and gel together until combined, and slowly stir in water until blended. Transfer to a small spray bottle and add in essential oil. To use, shake bottle and spritz sparingly throughout hair.

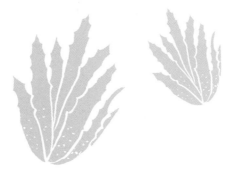

Volumizing Citrus Spray

 N/O

2 cups distilled water
1 teaspoon white sugar
Juice of ½ lemon
Juice of ½ orange

Keep your hair from falling flat with this easy-to-make, gentle-on-hair volumizing spray. This recipe works great as a styling product but also works wonders as a hair-refreshing tonic on days that your style has lost its volume but you don't have time to shampoo and restyle.

In a small saucepan, heat water over medium heat, and stir in sugar until dissolved. Strain juices so as to eliminate any pulp or seeds, and add to saucepan. Allow mixture to cool, and transfer to a spray bottle. To use, spritz sparingly on damp or dry hair, and style as usual.

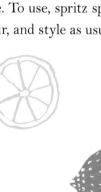

Split End-Mending Balm

N/D

2 tablespoons beeswax

1 teaspoon castor oil

½ teaspoon extra-virgin olive oil

Split ends are the bane of my existence. They are so unsightly and frustrating! Unfortunately, the only solution is to snip them, but this balm is great for temporarily sealing them and protecting your hair against future damage!

Melt beeswax in a double boiler set over medium heat, and stir in remaining oils, blending thoroughly. Pour balm into a resealable small tin, and let cool, uncovered, until hardened.

Use on dry hair, applying a small amount to ends.

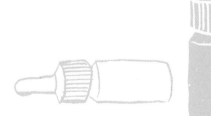

Aloe-Almond De-Frizzing Spray

N/D

1 cup distilled water
1 tablespoon aloe vera gel
1 tablespoon aloe vera juice
1 teaspoon almond oil

Frizzy hair is a major hair complaint of many women, and while there are tons of anti-frizz serums and sprays out there, many of them contain heavy silicones that weigh down hair, cause product buildup and are difficult to shampoo away. This spray eliminates frizz and keeps hair hydrated and nourished, and it's extremely easy to make.

Warm water in a small saucepan set over low heat. Remove from heat, and pour into an empty spray bottle. Before the water cools, combine remaining ingredients, close bottle and shake vigorously until ingredients are blended. Allow to cool before use.

To use, spritz onto damp hair before styling or onto dry hair to refresh and restyle. Store in a cool, dry place.

All-Natural Detangling Spray

ALL

2 cups distilled water
1 teaspoon aloe vera gel
1 teaspoon vegetable glycerine
$\frac{1}{2}$ teaspoon jojoba oil

Ripping through tangles is not only painful but can cause a lot of damage to your hair. If tangles are a problem for you, then this spray is a necessity for any hair-brushing session. This recipe is also perfect for kids.

Warm water in a small saucepan set over low heat. Remove from heat, and transfer into a spray bottle. Add remaining ingredients to the spray bottle, close the bottle, then shake vigorously. Allow to cool before use.

Spray on damp or dry hair before brushing.

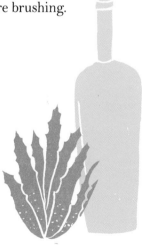

Volumizing Clay Hair Mask

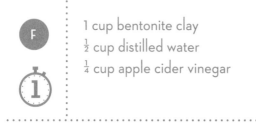

1 cup bentonite clay
½ cup distilled water
¼ cup apple cider vinegar

Clay masks are wonderful for skin, and they also work wonders to plump up and fortify your hair. Utilizing this mask just twice a month will give you a dramatic improvement in your hair's health and texture!

Stir ingredients together in a small bowl until a smooth paste forms. Massage into wet hair and leave on for 15 minutes. Rinse thoroughly, and condition.

Hair-Growth Serum

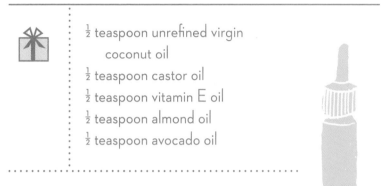

½ teaspoon unrefined virgin
    coconut oil
½ teaspoon castor oil
½ teaspoon vitamin E oil
½ teaspoon almond oil
½ teaspoon avocado oil

*Many of us lust after lengthy locks, and by now it's
pretty clear that the best route to mermaidlike hair is
by focusing on hair and scalp health. This serum deeply penetrates the
scalp and provides optimal health and nutrition for speedy hair
growth!*

Combine ingredients in a small bottle, and shake. Apply sparingly to dry scalp at night, using a Q-tip or a small brush to apply directly to the scalp. Shampoo or apply dry shampoo the next morning.

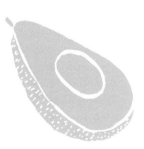

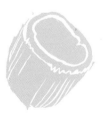

chapter 6

Body

. . . .

This chapter covers the biggest area of them all—the body! Most people are pretty conscientious about grooming and pampering their hair and face, but a lot of times the skin on the body gets overlooked. Break that habit by employing any (or all) of the scrubs, soaks, lotions and oils you'll find in this chapter. Your skin will be glowing in no time, and you'll realize how important it is to care for your body!

    I also love this chapter because there are so many gifting opportunities—everyone can benefit from a good scrub or lotion!

Cleansing Recipes

This section contains recipes for cleansing washes, scrubs and soaps, not to mention a deodorant that you can make at home (and it actually works)! Try a few of these recipes and you'll feel squeaky-clean but not stripped of your essential natural oils (trust me, you want those).

Hydrating Coconut Milk Body Wash

ALL

$\frac{1}{2}$ cup coconut milk

1 cup liquid castile soap

1 tablespoon liquefied coconut oil

1 teaspoon vitamin E oil

1 teaspoon vegetable glycerin

10 drops essential oil of your choice

High-quality, hydrating, store-bought body wash can be pricey, but you can make an incredibly hydrating and cleansing body wash at home for only a couple of bucks. This body wash smells delicious, and keeps skin hydrated all day.

Combine all ingredients in resealable container of your choice. Shake before each use.

Honey Body Wash

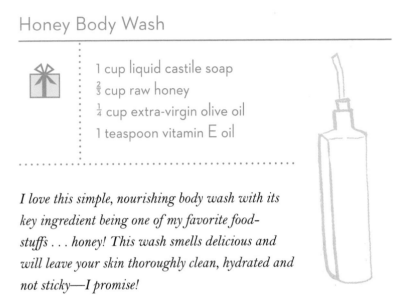

1 cup liquid castile soap

⅔ cup raw honey

¼ cup extra-virgin olive oil

1 teaspoon vitamin E oil

I love this simple, nourishing body wash with its key ingredient being one of my favorite foodstuffs . . . honey! This wash smells delicious and will leave your skin thoroughly clean, hydrated and not sticky—I promise!

Combine all ingredients in a squeeze bottle, and shake vigorously to thoroughly combine. Shake gently before each use.

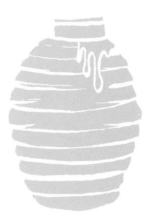

Citus Salt Scrub

½ cup sea salt
2 tablespoons extra-virgin olive oil
1 teaspoon unrefined virgin
    coconut oil
Zest of 1 lemon
Juice of ½ lemon

This body scrub is perfect for dull, dry skin; it effectively exfoliates even the most hardened of dry skin and then nourishes with deeply hydrating coconut and olive oils.

In resealable container of your choice, stir salt and oils together, ensuring the salt is thoroughly coated in oil before adding the citrus ingredients. Stir in remaining ingredients. To use, massage scrub all over dry skin in circular motions before showering.

Pit-Conditioning Deodorant

ALL

2 tablespoons unrefined virgin coconut oil

2 tablespoons raw shea butter

$\frac{1}{4}$ cup baking soda

$\frac{1}{4}$ cup arrowroot powder or cornstarch

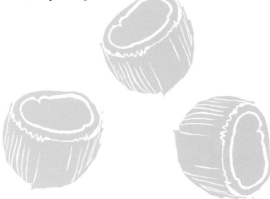

Un-fresh armpits and irritated armpits: Both are things that do not feel great, but often you can't relieve one without having the other. This homemade deodorant soothes and hydrates your sensitive pits while keeping unpleasant fragrances at bay.

Stir ingredients together in a small bowl. (I find that a fork is a really great tool for thoroughly stirring these ingredients together.) Store in a small, airtight container. To use, rub a small amount onto clean, dry armpits.

Strawberry Body Exfoliant

6 large strawberries with the tops removed, diced
1 tablespoon sugar
1 tablespoon honey
½ tablespoon unrefined virgin coconut oil
Juice of 1 lemon wedge

Strawberries are delicious little fruits full of exfoliating and hydrating power. With its namesake fruit, a touch of sugar and some seriously hydrating oil, this scrub will give you delectable skin that glows.

Mash strawberries in a bowl, and then stir in the remaining ingredients. Apply to dry skin and massage in circular motions for several minutes. Rinse thoroughly, and cleanse.

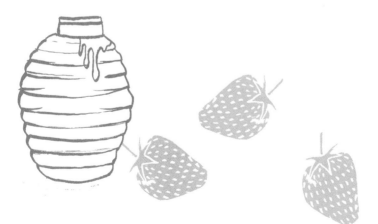

Orange-Ginger Foot Scrub

2 tablespoons unrefined virgin coconut oil

2 tablespoons sea salt

1 tablespoon freshly grated ginger

Zest of $\frac{1}{2}$ orange

This scrub invigorates and beautifies the roughest and most tired of feet. Orange exfoliates, while ginger stimulates and provides a wonderful, spicy fragrance. I recommend using this scrub at least once a week to pamper your tired dogs!

Stir oil and salt together until the salt is entirely coated with the oil. Melt the coconut oil mixture in the microwave first if necessary. Stir in the grated ginger and the zest of the orange and let "marinate" at least overnight in the fridge. Scrub onto dry heels, soles and ankles. Rinse thoroughly, and follow with lotion.

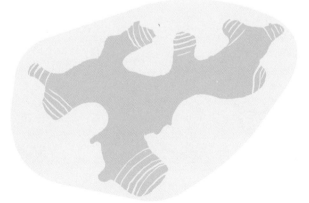

Foaming Body Wash for Acne-Prone Skin

O/A	2 cups distilled water

$\frac{1}{4}$ cup basil leaves

1 cup liquid castile soap

1 tablespoon jojoba oil

1 tablespoon vegetable glycerine

20 drops tea tree essential oil

Body acne, which can be caused by anything from stress and hormones to allergies and laundry detergent, is pretty frustrating. The best solution is to gently medicate, and exfoliate your skin every day. Use this body wash with a soft loofah and you'll soon see clearer skin from head to toe!

In a small saucepan, bring water to a boil. Remove from heat, toss in basil leaves and allow leaves to steep for at least 2 hours and up to overnight. After steeping, strain the leaves from the water, and combine water in a resealable bottle with remaining ingredients. Shake gently to combine.

To use, shake gently, apply a small amount to a wet loofah, lather and massage onto wet skin. Rinse thoroughly, and use daily.

Invigorating Coffee Scrub

¼ cup coffee grounds (it may sound odd, but you can even use used coffee grounds from your coffeemaker!)

¼ cup extra-virgin olive oil

2 tablespoons honey

2 tablespoons white sugar

A jolt of caffeine does wonders for a tired mind but also works miracles for dull or sagging skin. This scrub truly perks you up physically and mentally, and you'll see a marked difference in the tone and tightness of your skin after a few uses!

Stir ingredients together in a small bowl until thoroughly combined. Scrub onto dry skin before showering, and massage in circular motions for about 2 minutes. Rinse thoroughly, and cleanse.

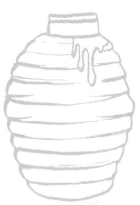

Moisturizing Recipes

It's most important to moisturize the skin on our bodies—the skin is much thicker there than on the face, and it has far less naturally moisturizing oil glands, so it tends to dry out much more quickly. Be sure to use a body lotion or cream on a daily basis and a moisturizing scrub regularly!

Mango Body Butter

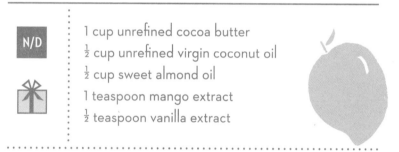

N/D

1 cup unrefined cocoa butter
½ cup unrefined virgin coconut oil
½ cup sweet almond oil
1 teaspoon mango extract
½ teaspoon vanilla extract

This recipe is an all-natural interpretation of a former store-bought favorite that I discovered contained some rather unsavory ingredients. This body butter is hydrating, smells super delicious and makes a wonderful gift!

Melt cocoa butter and coconut oil in a double boiler set over medium heat. Remove from heat, and stir in almond oil, mango extract and vanilla extract. Let chill in the fridge for 2 hours, or until the mixture begins to solidify. Remove from the fridge and whip with a hand mixer until a consistent whipped texture has been reached. Transfer to a resealable glass jar, and let cool thoroughly before using.

Olive Oil and Rose Bath Soak

ALL	¼ cup extra-virgin olive oil
	½ cup rose water
	20 drops rose essential oil

A soak in a hot bath has truly transformative effects on the mind and body. This decadent soak is a wonderful way to relax and hydrate the skin. Olive oil hydrates and conditions while rose pampers and calms your mind. This recipe makes one soak, but you can mix up a larger batch and store it in a cool, dry place.

Combine ingredients and pour them into running bathwater. For extra luxuriousness, sprinkle fresh rose petals into the tub. (Don't forget an accompanying flute of champagne!) Soak for 30 minutes or as long as you desire.

Hydrating Body Oil

N/D

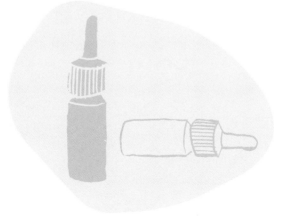

$\frac{1}{4}$ cup sesame oil

$\frac{1}{4}$ cup sweet almond oil

1 tablespoon vitamin E oil

10 drops essential oil of your choice (if desired)

Using body oil is a wonderful and lightweight way to deliver deep hydration while adding a beautiful glow to the skin. Not only is creating body oil super easy, but you'll see a drastic difference in the moisture and radiance of your skin after just the first use.

Combine ingredients in resealable container of your choice. I personally prefer pump dispensers (a repurposed body lotion bottle works great), as they are the least messy. Shake gently. To use, massage a small amount onto clean skin after a bath or shower.

Skin-Smoothing Shaving Cream

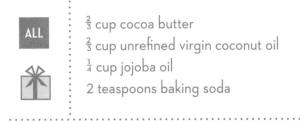

⅔ cup cocoa butter

⅔ cup unrefined virgin coconut oil

¼ cup jojoba oil

2 teaspoons baking soda

Shaving is a great way to achieve smooth skin. Obviously, it rids the body of excess hair, but it also lightly exfoliates, which allows lotions, creams or oils to penetrate the skin more easily. This recipe is similar to the Mango Body Butter recipe (page 135) but with a few tweaks that make it easier to use with a razor. It prepares the skin for shaving and does half the work of your body lotion or oil.

In a double boiler, melt cocoa butter and coconut oil over medium heat. Remove from heat and stir in jojoba oil. Let chill in the fridge until solidified. Remove from fridge, and let sit at room temperature for about 5 minutes. Stir in baking soda, and whip mixture with a hand mixer until liquefied. Transfer to resealable container of your choice.

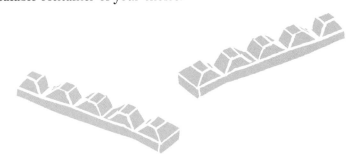

Almond-Rose Body Lotion

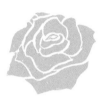

¾ cup sweet almond oil

2 tablespoons beeswax

1 cup rose water

30 drops rose essential oil

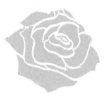

This supremely hydrating lotion not only deeply nourishes but also helps your skin retain moisture all day long. The luxurious rose fragrance makes you feel pampered and beautiful. This is another recipe that makes a great gift when it's packaged in a pretty glass jar.

Combine the sweet almond oil and beeswax in a double boiler over low to medium heat until the beeswax liquefies.

Pour the rose water into a blender and put the lid on but keep the hole for pouring in liquids open. Start blending on high and then slowly pour the oil combo into the blender through the lid hole. Once the mixture thickens, stop blending and stir in the rose essential oil.

For best results, slather this luxurious lotion on right after you step out of the shower.

Soothing Lavender-Eucalyptus Massage Oil

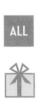

1 cup extra-virgin olive oil
2 tablespoons castor oil
15 drops lavender essential oil
10 drops eucalyptus essential oil

I love giving, and especially receiving, massages, and when you're really serious about performing some relaxing touch, a normal lotion simply won't do. This oil gives great slip—but not too much, so that

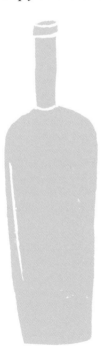

you still have control over your movements, rather than sliding all over the place. Lavender and eucalyptus are my favorite scents for massage oil; lavender makes me feel very relaxed while eucalyptus soothes sore muscles and joints. That said, you can experiment with your favorite essential oils to come up with your own custom-blended massage oil!

Combine all ingredients in a bottle, and shake gently to combine. Use on clean, dry skin. Rinse if desired (though not necessary).

Shake before each use, and store in a cool, dry place.

Lavender Hand Cream

ALL

2 tablespoons beeswax
2 tablespoons cocoa butter
2 tablespoons shea butter
1 teaspoon sweet almond oil
15 drops lavender essential oil

Hand cream is one of those items that is hugely beneficial to use but oftentimes goes overlooked. This recipe makes a hydrating, soothing and protective hand cream that helps you pamper yourself throughout the day and makes a really nice gift.

Combine beeswax and cocoa and shea butters in a double boiler set over medium heat until melted. Remove from heat and stir in almond and lavender essential oils. Let chill in the fridge until partially solidified. Remove and whip with a hand mixer until desired consistency is reached. Transfer hand cream to a resealable small jar or tin for storage.

Lavender

Lavender is widely revered for its calming and soothing effects on mood, and it also soothes skin topically. Believe it or not, lavender also has antifungal and antiseptic characteristics, which are wonderful for the health of skin (lavender can actually expedite healing) and hair.

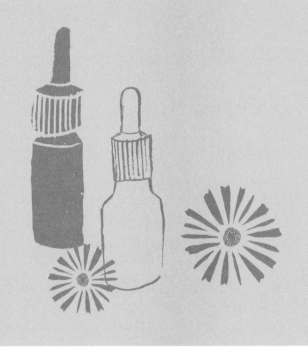

Peppermint-Vanilla Foot Cream

$\frac{1}{4}$ cup cocoa butter

2 tablespoons unrefined virgin coconut oil

$\frac{1}{2}$ teaspoon vanilla extract

15 drops peppermint essential oil

Foot cream is yet another "accessory cream" that often goes unused but is really lovely and extremely beneficial once you get into the habit of using it. This recipe in particular is decadent and refreshing, and its scent makes it the perfect holiday gift!

Melt cocoa butter and coconut oil in a double boiler set over low to medium heat. Remove from heat, and stir in vanilla extract and peppermint essential oil. Let chill in the fridge until partially solidified. Remove and whip with a hand mixer until desired consistency is reached (I prefer a thicker foot cream). Transfer to your desired container.

For best results, slather onto clean feet before bed. Put on a pair of socks and allow your feet to soak up the cream overnight!

Olive Oil Skin Salve

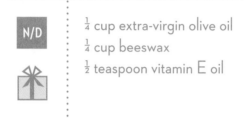

¼ cup extra-virgin olive oil

¼ cup beeswax

½ teaspoon vitamin E oil

Salves are great for rough patches of skin, cuts, scrapes, bruises and blemishes that are on the mend. This recipe hydrates and protects, allowing for speedy healing!

Combine ingredients in a double boiler set over low to medium heat, until melted. Remove from heat, transfer to a resealable tin or salve container of your choice and let cool before placing the lid on the container.

To use, apply generously to desired areas.

Homemade Lotion Bars

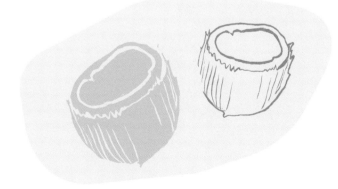

¾ cup beeswax
¼ cup shea butter
¼ cup unrefined virgin coconut oil
20 drops essential oil of your choice
6 to 8 soap molds

Lotion bars are amazing for traveling; they are a completely leak-free way to moisturize your skin on the go. The recipe is similar to many of the lotion recipes in the book, made with just a little more beeswax and formed into a beautiful mold!

Melt all solid ingredients in a double boiler until liquefied. Remove from heat, stir in essential oil and allow mixture to cool slightly. Pour liquid evenly into molds and allow to harden—this should take about 2 hours. Pop your solidified lotion out of the molds and voilà! Lotion bars!

To use, rub over clean, dry skin. Do not rinse.

Body-Glow Oil

½ cup sweet almond oil
1 tablespoon castor oil
1 tablespoon silver mica powder
½ tablespoon zinc oxide powder

When the season allows us to expose some skin, there's nothing more beautiful than hydrated, glowing skin. This body-glow oil not only moisturizes the skin but "cheats" a little bit with some light-reflecting particles. Slather this on arms and legs before a night out and you'll be glowing all night long!

Combine all ingredients in a resealable glass bottle. Shake to combine. Shake before each use and apply to clean, dry skin.

Coconut-Shea Sunscreen

$\frac{1}{4}$ cup unrefined virgin coconut oil

$\frac{1}{4}$ cup shea butter

2 tablespoons jojoba oil

1 teaspoon vitamin E oil

2 tablespoons zinc oxide powder

It's so important to protect our skin from the damaging rays of the sun. We all know overexposure to the sun can lead to skin cancer, and it is also the number one cause of premature aging. Did you know that just a sunburn can cause wrinkles that don't start appearing for another five years?

To be totally honest, most sunscreens on the market are full of toxic and harmful chemicals; plus they do a great job of clogging pores and making your skin feel really greasy and gross. This all-natural formula is totally healthy and protects the skin while hydrating and nourishing.

Melt coconut oil and shea butter in a double boiler set over low to medium heat until liquefied. Remove from heat, and stir in remaining ingredients while still hot. Pour into desired container, and let cool.

To use, massage all over skin before sun exposure. Reapply every hour or so.

Coconut-Lemon-Sugar Body Scrub

ALL

¼ cup unrefined virgin coconut oil
2 tablespoons coconut milk
¼ cup sugar
1 teaspoon lemon juice
1 tablespoon lemon zest

Delicious, hydrating and refreshing, this scrub is perfect for achieving that luxurious glow. I especially love using this in the summer—the coconut scent takes my mind directly to the beach.

Melt the coconut oil in a double boiler over low heat or in the microwave on medium for 15 to 20 seconds, and stir in coconut milk and sugar, mixing until the sugar is thoroughly coated. Stir in lemon juice and lemon zest until all ingredients are combined. Transfer to a glass jar.

To use, massage all over dry skin before showering. Rinse thoroughly, and cleanse.

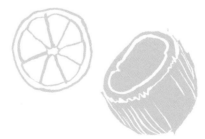

Lemon Cuticle Cream

1 tablespoon shea butter
1 tablespoon grated beeswax
1 tablespoon unrefined virgin
   coconut oil
10 drops lemon essential oil

From hand washing to cold weather, our delicate cuticles are the first place on our hands that take a beating. Keep your cuticles soft and protected with this hydrating, fresh cream.

Melt shea butter, beeswax and coconut oil in a double boiler set over medium heat. Remove from heat, and stir in lemon essential oil. Pour into a small resealable tin and allow to fully cool before covering with the lid.

To use, massage a small amount into cuticles daily.

Soothing Oatmeal Bath

N/D

①

1 clean sock or coffee filter
1 rubber band
¾ cup plain rolled oats
2 tablespoons unrefined virgin coconut oil

This soak is perfect for anyone who suffers from psoriasis or eczema, or for anyone whose skin is feeling itchy, irritated, dry or tight. It's a fast, easy and effective fix!

Pour oatmeal into sock or coffee filter and close off with a rubber band. Put "sachet" into the bathtub and run yourself a hot bath. Once your bath has been drawn, stir in coconut oil. Soak in soothing oatmeal bath for at least 15 minutes.

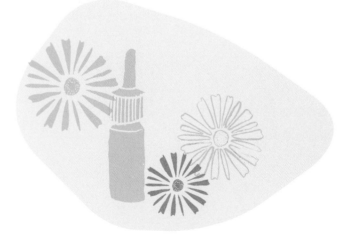

Ingredient Spotlight

Oatmeal

When moistened, oatmeal forms a nourishing paste that, applied topically, hydrates and protects the skin. Oatmeal also cleanses pores of dirt and impurities. It's great combined with other skin-loving ingredients, but even oatmeal applied alone will work wonders on your skin.

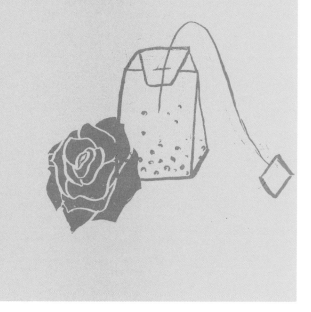

Brown Sugar–Vanilla Body Scrub

N/D

2 cups brown sugar
½ cup extra-virgin olive oil
½ cup honey
1 tablespoon vanilla extract

This scrub not only sloughs off dead cells but also deeply hydrates the skin, giving a gorgeous glow! This is a recipe that I have a hard time not eating with a spoon . . . the ingredients are a tad difficult to resist! It makes an impressive, beautiful gift—nobody will know how inexpensive it was to make, because it looks just like the $30 version sold at high-end spas!

Mix ingredients until there are no lumps, and get to scrubbing, focusing on knees, elbows and heels. Rinse thoroughly.

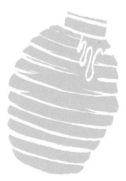

Detoxifying Recipes

From your diet to your environment, your body encounters numerous toxins on a day-to-day basis. This can make your skin look dull, clog your pores and make you feel sluggish. Treat yourself to a detoxifying treatment several times a month, and you'll notice that your skin glows!

Invigorating Matcha-Green Tea Bath Soak

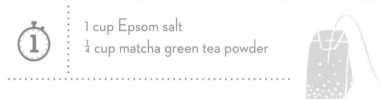

1 cup Epsom salt

$\frac{1}{4}$ cup matcha green tea powder

Matcha green tea powder is basically like concentrated green tea. It's full of antioxidants, makes delicious drinks and also makes an incredible rejuvenating bath soak. Be warned, however, that this recipe will give you a jolt of energy, so it is best for mornings or afternoons. It also tints your bathwater a pale green color, which I personally think is a lot of fun. This recipe is enough for a single serving, but you can mix up a larger batch and store it for more soaks!

Combine ingredients, and pour them under running water into a hot bath. Soak for at least 15 minutes.

Impurity-Dissolving Body Soak

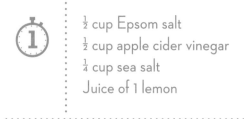

½ cup Epsom salt

½ cup apple cider vinegar

¼ cup sea salt

Juice of 1 lemon

This treatment isn't the most posh or glamorous, but it is sure to draw out toxins and impurities from the body and make you feel like a whole new person.

Draw a bath as hot as you can stand and add in all ingredients, stirring until ingredients are dissolved, and soak for 30 minutes. Be sure to get out of the tub slowly (you may be a little light-headed from this detoxifying soak), and drink plenty of water after you're done, to avoid dehydration.

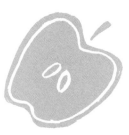

Ginger-Lemon Oxygen Bath

(1)

1 cup hydrogen peroxide
¼ cup freshly grated ginger
Juice of 1 lemon

When hydrogen peroxide is used in a soak, it's often referred to as an "oxygen bath," which not only sounds awesome but will make you feel incredible. Hydrogen helps to rid the body of toxins, and when you combine that with blood flow–stimulating ginger and antioxidant-rich lemon, you have a super-effective detox soak.

Draw a bath as hot as you can stand and add all ingredients, stirring to blend, and soak for 30 minutes. Be sure to drink a lot of water afterward to replenish what you sweat out!

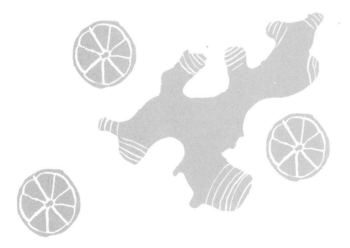

Detoxifying Mud Body Mask

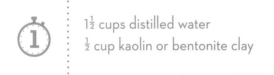

1½ cups distilled water
½ cup kaolin or bentonite clay

Clay-based "muds" are a super-effective and safe way of decongesting pores. This treatment pulls toxins out of your skin and gives your body a beautiful glow. Not to mention it is really messy . . . in a fun way!

Heat water in a medium saucepan until it reaches a comfortable temperature. Slowly pour water into clay, stirring continuously, and stop when it's reached a pasty, mudlike texture. In the tub, massage treatment all over your body (you can use it head to toe!). Let sit for at least 5 minutes, or for best results, soak in a hot bath for up to 15 minutes. Rinse off thoroughly in the shower.

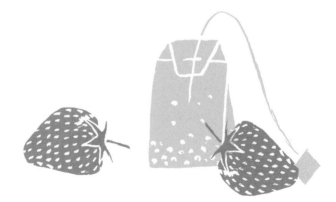

Detoxifying Rosemary Foot Soak

$\frac{3}{4}$ cup Epsom salt

$\frac{1}{4}$ cup sea salt

$\frac{1}{4}$ cup baking soda

$\frac{1}{4}$ cup dried rosemary leaves

20 drops essential oil of your choice (I prefer lavender)

If your feet are tired and you're feeling sluggish, this recipe is for you. Epsom salt and rosemary leaves soothe sore muscles, while baking soda provides a detoxifying cleanse. This soak makes an incredible gift and is perfect for friends and family members who are on their feet for most of the day! This recipe makes 1 "serving," but you can mix up a larger batch for a gift or for your own personal storage.

Place all ingredients in a large mixing bowl, and stir to combine. Pour water as hot as your feet can stand into a large bowl or basin and stir in salt mixture. Allow feet to soak for 30 minutes. Rinse thoroughly, and cleanse.

Dead Skin-Dissolving Foot Treatment

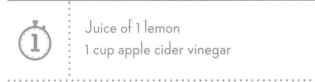

Juice of 1 lemon
1 cup apple cider vinegar

Stubborn callouses on your feet can be difficult to remove. Luckily, this treatment does half the work for you. Allow your feet to soak in this before you go at them with a pumice stone and you'll see noticeably smoother feet.

Fill a basin or large bowl with hot water and add lemon juice and vinegar. Soak feet for 15 minutes, and then follow immediately with an exfoliating pumice stone or scrub. Rinse thoroughly, and cleanse.

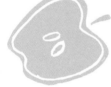

Red Wine Antioxidant Bath

4 cups red wine
2 tablespoons unrefined virgin coconut oil

This soak is super decadent (hello . . . it's primarily red wine) and a lot of fun. Not only that, but it is one of the most antioxidizing treatments you can use. Red wine is full of antioxidants, skin-

preserving polyphenols and exfoliating tartaric acid. Don't worry, you don't need to waste any high-quality red wine on this . . . any type of red wine will do!

Add ingredients to a hot bath and swirl to blend. Allow yourself to soak for at least 15 minutes. Rinse thoroughly, and cleanse.

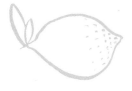

Anti-Cellulite Ginger Scrub

$\frac{1}{2}$ cup sugar
2 tablespoons unrefined virgin coconut oil
2 tablespoons grated fresh ginger
Juice of 1 lemon

I won't lie and tell you that a scrub alone can get rid of your cellulite, but with a little manual motivation and some exercise, you can certainly reduce the appearance of unwanted bumps. This invigorating scrub increases blood flow to areas with cellulite, which in turn helps the body smooth things out.

Combine sugar and coconut oil in a bowl until sugar is completely coated. Stir in remaining ingredients and mix thoroughly. On dry skin, massage vigorously and with circular motions onto areas of concern for about 2 minutes. Rinse thoroughly, and cleanse.

Pampering Recipes

The pampering recipes for the body are the most decadent of them all; from soaks, baths, scrubs and treatments, you're sure to feel super luxurious. On the other hand, some of these recipes are for pampering your ailments—razor burn, sunburn and insect bites. No matter what your ailment, if you treat it naturally, you're sure to recover in no time!

Chamomile-Mint Bath Soak

6 bags chamomile tea or 6
    tablespoons loose chamomile tea
$\frac{1}{4}$ cup mint leaves, de-stemmed
1 clean sock or coffee filter
1 rubber band

Sometimes you just need to unwind, and one of the best natural resources for relaxation is chamomile. Combine that with cooling mint and you'll be chilled out in no time! This recipe gives you a relaxing bath sachet and, when packaged beautifully (hint: I wouldn't use the sock), makes a great gift.

If using tea bags, cut bags open and pour the contents into sock or coffee filter. Add mint leaves, and secure "sachet" with rubber band. Toss in the tub and run a hot bath. Soak for at least 15 minutes.

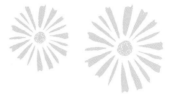

Muscle-Healing Salt Scrub

ALL

½ cup Epsom salt

¼ cup sea salt

¼ cup extra-virgin olive oil

10 drops peppermint essential oil

10 drops eucalyptus essential oil

Sore muscles are a great sign that you got an efficient workout, but they are also incredibly distracting and painful! This scrub soothes away any aches and pains post-workout and, as an added bonus, gives your skin a beautiful glow.

Stir ingredients together until a consistent texture has been reached. On dry skin, gently massage onto sore muscles for a few minutes. Rinse and cleanse.

You can also eliminate the olive oil and sea salt and add the remaining ingredients to a hot bath for a soothing soak.

Peppermint-Tea Tree Invigorating Foot Soak

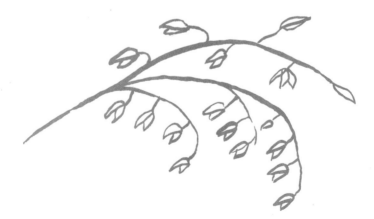

½ cup Epsom salt
¼ cup baking soda
10 drops peppermint essential oil
10 drops tea tree essential oil

Tired, achey feet can put a damper on your entire mood. This soak is a great treat for overworked feet and will definitely brighten you up. Peppermint oil and tea tree oil perk you up and awaken the senses, while Epsom salt soothes aches.

Fill a large bowl or basin with hot water and add all ingredients, stirring to combine. Allow your feet to soak for at least 15 minutes.

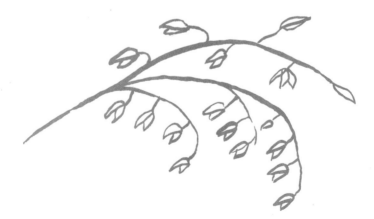

Rose-Grapefruit Body Spray

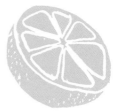

1 cup distilled water
1 tablespoon witch hazel
1 teaspoon vitamin E oil
10 drops grapefruit essential oil
10 drops rose essential oil

I love the luxurious feeling of spritzing on a refreshing scented body spray. Most body sprays are filled with irritating alcohol and tons of chemicals, but this all-natural version will keep you fresh and healthy.

Combine ingredients in a spray bottle and shake gently to combine. Spritz onto your body wherever and whenever you want a pick-me-up!

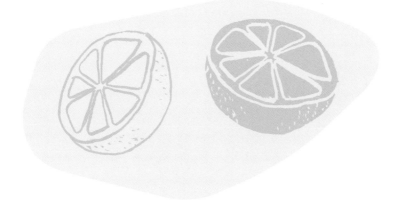

Peppermint Lotion for Soothing Sore Muscles

⅓ cup beeswax

½ cup shea butter

½ cup unrefined virgin coconut oil

15 drops peppermint essential oil

10 drops eucalyptus essential oil

Besides not having aches in the first place, can you think of anything better for sore muscles than a gentle massage with cooling and soothing lotion? I don't think so. This lotion hydrates the skin and relieves pain and discomfort.

Melt beeswax, shea butter and coconut oil on low heat in a double boiler. Remove from heat and stir in essential oils. Allow to cool in the fridge until solidified. Remove from fridge, and whip with a hand mixer until desired consistency is reached. To use, gently massage onto clean, dry skin. Store in a cool, dry place.

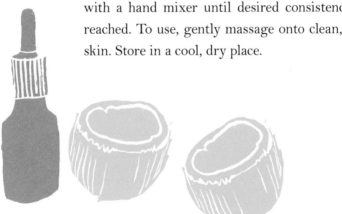

Soothing Summer Body Spray

ALL

1 cup distilled water
1 tablespoon aloe vera gel
1 tablespoon unrefined virgin coconut oil
½ cup aloe vera juice

Summer is my favorite season, but that doesn't particularly mean it's the most comfortable. From sunburns to heat rash to just feeling flat-out overheated, sometimes you need something to soothe and cool your skin. This recipe makes the perfect spray to keep in your beach or pool bag for refreshing on the go! It also gives skin a beautiful glow.

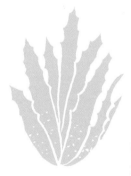

In a small saucepan, heat water over low to medium heat for 5 minutes. Add aloe vera gel and coconut oil, and stir until both have melted into the water. Remove from heat and stir in aloe vera juice. Allow to fully cool, and then transfer to a spray bottle. Shake to combine. Store in a cool, dry place or chill in the fridge for the most refreshing of sprays!

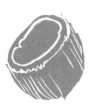

Cooling Anti-Itch Treatment

2 tablespoons baking soda
½ cup distilled water
Juice of ½ lemon
5 drops peppermint essential oil

This cream works wonders for bug bites, rashes and any type of itchy, irritated skin. This batch is for one-time use only, but luckily it's super easy to whip up, so you can have it ready at a moment's notice!

Stir ingredients together until a paste forms. Apply to affected areas and allow to dry. Rinsing is optional.

Eucalyptus Bug-Repellent Spray

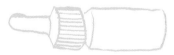

1 teaspoon eucalyptus essential oil
1 tablespoon castor oil
¼ cup witch hazel
½ cup distilled water

Most bug-repellent sprays are chock-full of extremely harmful and irritating chemicals. This recipe can be used anywhere, on anyone, and will not cause any inflammation, respiratory problems or any other consequences that spraying yourself with chemicals might have!

Combine ingredients in a spray bottle. Mist exposed skin before heading outdoors. Re-apply every hour or so.

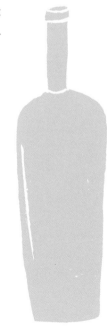

After-Sun Aloe Treatment

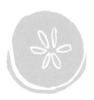

¼ cup aloe vera gel
1 cucumber, peeled and diced
20 drops lavender essential oil

I love spending time in the sun, but it's safe to say that we've all overstayed our outdoor welcome before and gotten a bit too sun-kissed. I definitely recommend avoiding overexposure to the sun as much as possible (it can lead to premature aging even years after the actual exposure), but if you come home looking akin to a lobster, definitely treat yourself with this after-sun concoction.

Place aloe vera gel and cucumber in a blender, and blend on low until smooth. Stir in lavender essential oil. Massage into affected areas. Rinsing is optional.

Tea Tree Oil Razor Burn Treatment

ALL

1 tablespoon jojoba oil
2 tablespoons unrefined virgin coconut oil
1 teaspoon tea tree essential oil

The purpose of shaving, from what I can tell, is to achieve smooth, flawless skin. Razor burn is the visual antithesis of this, and beyond frustrating! This treatment eliminates razor burn and keeps your skin smooth and soft.

Melt coconut oil in double boiler over low heat. Stir all ingredients together until thoroughly blended. To use, apply generously onto clean, dry skin directly after shaving.

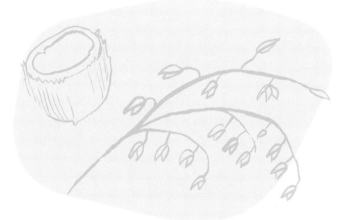

Indulgent Chocolate Bath

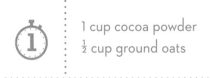

1 cup cocoa powder
½ cup ground oats

I'm a self-confessed chocoholic, so imagine my joy when I discovered how beneficial chocolate is to the skin. It rids the body of toxins, improves circulation and boosts hydration! It's also proven to elevate mood. This recipe makes 1 bath treatment, but you can mix up a larger batch for gifting or for your own personal storage.

Add ingredients to a hot bath and stir to distribute. Soak for at least 20 minutes. After soaking, rinse thoroughly.

Body Powder

1 cup arrowroot powder or cornstarch
20 drops essential oil of your choice (blend up to
   3 different oils)

*A lot of people don't think to use body powders, but they can work
wonders during summer's stickier months. I love applying a body
powder on areas where I tend to sweat more, and it keeps me super
comfortable and smelling great!*

Slowly drip essential oil into cornstarch while stirring
continuously, until there are no clumps. Store in a
shaker jar (like the ones intended for Parmesan
cheese or red pepper flakes). Apply to clean, dry
skin after showering.

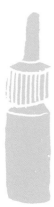
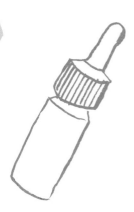

Custom-Blended Perfume

ALL

¼ cup 100 proof vodka

3 of your favorite essential oils

Store-bought perfumes are loaded with harmful chemicals, and when you buy a mass-produced scent, you run the risk of smelling like millions of other people. I love creating my own signature scent by custom-blending my own perfume. What's great is that it takes only two ingredients and a little creativity. The only tricky part here is finding the best blend of essential oils. Personally, I love floral blends, so I find myself using a lot of lavender, rose, and ylang ylang essential oil with a deeper base note such as patchouli or sandalwood. This is a great recipe to use when you have some friends over (or during a bridal or baby shower) and want to partake in a fun group activity.

In a small glass container or spray bottle, combine vodka and 20 or so drops of each essential oil. Again, it's going to take some trial and error finding the best blends and ratios of essential oils, but that's the fun in creating your own scent!

Olive Oil and Lemon Nail Strengthener

ALL

1 tablespoon extra-virgin olive oil
1 tablespoon vitamin E oil
20 drops lemon essential oil

Brittle, flaky and thin nails are no fun, even if you prefer your nails short . . . They're even less fun if you prefer sporting longer talons. This oil works wonders for strengthening your nails and hydrating your cuticles, and you'll see a dramatic difference after just a few uses!

Combine all ingredients in a small glass bottle and shake to combine. Apply several times a day using a Q-tip, and massage into nails and cuticles.

Ingredient Spotlight
Olive Oil

O live oil is something we've all probably used and consumed for the majority of our lives. You won't even believe how thrilled I was when I discovered how incredible it is for topical use on hair, skin, body and nails—I could (and sometimes do) bathe in the stuff! Extra-virgin olive oil is fantastic because it is full of vitamins E and A, which moisturize and plump the skin and hair. Small amounts are easily absorbed into skin and hair, but don't overdo it! When used too generously, olive oil can make your hair and skin greasy.

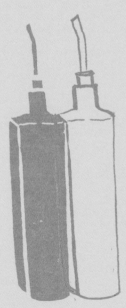

Mint-Aloe Cooling Foot Spray

1 cup distilled water
$\frac{1}{4}$ cup aloe vera juice
$\frac{1}{4}$ cup witch hazel
20 drops peppermint essential oil

When it's hot outside or when you have days spent entirely on your feet, there's nothing more refreshing than a cooling and relaxing foot treatment. Unfortunately, you don't always have the time or the space to do a full-on foot soak, which is where this foot spray comes in. This product is especially handy to keep in your gym bag, to use after yoga classes or if you have a house where shoes aren't allowed inside . . . it has fabulous deodorizing capabilities!

Combine all ingredients in a spray bottle and shake to combine. Spray onto dry feet whenever you like!

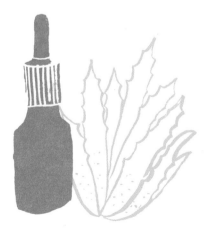

Resources

Guide to Essential Oils

CLARY SAGE—Essential oil of clary sage is ideal for dry skin and oily skin and for combatting wrinkles. It's also great for speeding up hair growth.

GERANIUM—Geranium essential oil is useful for all skin types and can be implemented into any skincare routine. It's also hydrating for dry hair and enhances hair growth.

LAVENDER—Lavender essential oil is also useful for all skin types and all hair types; it's soothing and calming.

LEMON—Lemon is an uplifting essential oil that works wonders for fighting fungus, in addition to stimulating the immune system. It is also anti-inflammatory.

PEPPERMINT—Peppermint oil is beneficial for oily skin and hair.

ROSE—Rose essential oil is wonderful for calming nerves and gives a beautiful glow to skin and hair.

SANDALWOOD—Sandalwood is another essential oil that's beneficial for dry, oily and wrinkle-prone skin and helps hydrate dry hair. Sandalwood essential oil has a luxurious, rich fragrance.

TEA TREE—Tea tree works to zap zits, keep oil of the face and scalp at bay and rid your scalp of dandruff. Its scent is invigorating and clean.

YLANG YLANG—Ylang ylang essential oil improves firmness and elasticity of the skin, in addition to supporting healthy hair growth.

Guide to Carrier Oils

"Carrier oils" are low- to no-fragrance, non-evaporating oils that are used to dilute essential oils. For the purposes of this book, they also make great bases for scrubs and creams.

AVOCADO OIL—Avocados are a staple in many of our diets, but a lot of people overlook avocado oil, which has just as many hair and skin benefits as the fruit it comes from. Avocado oil moisturizes and volumizes mature or dry skin and hair. It contains proteins, omega-3 fatty acids and antioxidants that hydrate and plump the skin, increase collagen production and can help heal skin conditions and inflammation.

CASTOR OIL—Containing minerals, vitamin E and omega-6s, castor oil can stimulate hair growth, strengthen hair and help heal scalp conditions in addition to reducing inflammation and wrinkles. Used by itself, castor oil can sometimes make the skin feel dry, so it's nice to mix it with another carrier oil such as avocado oil or sweet almond oil.

COCONUT OIL—Coconut oil is seen in a number of recipes in this book because it's considered skin- and hair-care gold. It soothes irritation, penetrates the skin and hydrates deeply, fills in wrinkles and strengthens and moisturizes hair. In a pinch, I'll use it as a body moisturizer, face moisturizer and makeup remover. Be sure to purchase organic, raw, refined virgin coconut oil.

JOJOBA OIL—Jojoba oil is also suitable for all skin types but is especially beneficial for those with oily skin, due to the fact that jojoba most closely resembles our natural sebum. Thus, when applied, this oil sends signals to the oil glands to halt production. Jojoba can also help with enlarged pores and improve the health of scalp and hair.

OLIVE OIL—Suitable for all skin types, olive oil moisturizes, antioxidizes and is perfect for exfoliating when combined with an abrasive ingredient because it doesn't clog pores. Make sure to use high-quality, extra-virgin olive oil.

SUNFLOWER SEED OIL—Rich in vitamin E, sunflower seed oil is lightweight and protective. This oil actually works wonders on acne-prone skin: Apply several drops to clean skin to keep the skin protected from harmful bacteria.

SWEET ALMOND OIL—Almond oil is hydrating and firming for dry or mature skin. It's full of vitamins E and D, magnesium and calcium. Almond oil stimulates hair growth, strengthens hair, prevents aging and is even known to help with dark under-eye circles.

Creating Beautiful Packaging for Your Homemade Beauty Products

While some of the recipes found in *Homemade Beauty* are intended for one-time use only, many of them actually have quite a lengthy shelf life, making them not only worth the time and effort to create but also making them easily giftable.

Gifting homemade beauty products is incredibly thoughtful— not only are you giving the recipient a beauty product comparable to one of spa quality, but you are making it completely evident how much thought you are putting into the present. It doesn't get much sweeter than that.

I love making products for my friends who are beauty junkies, for loved ones who are suffering skin or hair ailments that may be remedied by my concoctions, or for those who need a little extra pampering but aren't so good about taking time for themselves to do so. In most cases, the recipients of my gifts ask for seconds or ask for other varieties of my homemade products; it creates a really fun relationship, and it feels really good to give.

While using recycled product bottles is a great and environmentally friendly idea for your personal homemade beauty products (just be sure to wash them thoroughly with warm water and soap before reusings), you may want to try something a little fancier or more creative when you're gifting your creations.

Hardware stores sell a wide variety of Mason jars, and stores like the Container Store sell beautiful hermetic jars that will seal your products airtight, which is fantastic for extending the shelf life of homemade beauty products. You can also find countless decorative jars and bottles at thrift stores, again, being sure to wash before use. When it comes to spray bottles and squeeze bottles, those can be found at beauty-supply stores and, again, the Container Store. Muji also stocks tons of well-designed pump bottles, spray bottles and jars, which you can also find in their online store.

You'll also want to label your gifts, and there are a number of creative and aesthetically pleasing ways to do so. If you have nice handwriting, you can create your own personal label with a sticker or on a tag attached with ribbon or twine (you can find decorative tags at craft stores and online). If labeling is not for you, you can always gift your product with a nice card explaining what it is and how/when to use it.

If you prefer a graphic design label, there are a ton of great websites where you can design your own jar and bottle labels. My personal favorite site is myownlabels.com, which has a ton of templates for labels that are inexpensive and easy to make. If you're lucky enough to be handy with Photoshop or any design software, obviously you can create a number of beautiful labels for your products. On the labels you can include just the product name, or include the ingredients as well!

The point is that you don't have to do anything fancy (or you can if you want to!). These thoughtful, lovingly made gifts speak for themselves.

All-Natural Beauty Brands I Love

Obviously, we can make pretty much any beauty product that we want at home, but I also still really enjoy seeing what's on the market and having something to compare my homemade goods to. A lot of these brands were also huge inspirations for my recipes and for branching out into homemade products in the first place. I definitely recommend you check these brands out and learn more about each brand's philosophy!

Alba Botanica
Aubrey Organics
Avalon Organics
Blades Natural Beauty
Earth Tu Face
Fat and the Moon
ILIA Beauty
Intelligent Nutrients
John Masters
    Organics

Living Libations
LuLu Organics
Pratima
REN Clean Skincare
RMS
SkinnySkinny
Soapwalla
Tata Harper

Acknowledgments

First and foremost, thank you to all the women who have opened up to me, shared their stories and inspired me to continue to pursue the beauty industry.

Thank you to my team at Lovelyish.com, my agent and my editor for such amazing opportunities and for your endless support.

I can't even fully express my appreciation for my family, especially my dad, who always encouraged me to find my passion despite myself; my mom, who taught me to keep laughing and my sister for seeing something in me that I still don't quite see myself.

My biggest thanks goes to my husband, who tirelessly cares for me and constantly finds ways to make my life easier. Without him, this book would not be possible.

Index

acne-prone skin. *See* oily and acne-prone skin
After-Sun Aloe Treatment, 168
After-Sun Hydrating Hair Treatment, 91
almond oil: about, 139, 180
  Almond-Rose Body Lotion, 139
  Aloe-Almond De-Frizzing Spray, 122
aloe vera
  After-Sun Aloe Treatment, 168
  Aloe-Almond De-Frizzing Spray, 122
  Avocado-Aloe Shampoo, 81
  De-Puffing Cucumber-Aloe Eye Gel, 60
  Lemon-Aloe Oil-Reducing Rinse, 104
  Mint-Aloe Cooling Foot Spray, 175
Anti-Acne Baking Soda Mask, 49
anti-aging treatments
  Anti-Aging Pumpkin Puree Mask, 46
  Carrot-Avocado Anti-Aging Mask, 41
  Firming Peach Mask, 40
  Skin-Tightening Egg White Mask, 39
Anti-Cellulite Ginger Scrub, 159
Anti-Itch Treatment, Cooling, 166
Antioxidant Bath, Red Wine, 158–59
apple cider vinegar: about, 6, 109
  Apple Cider Vinegar and Lemon Hair Rinse, 108
  Apple Cider Vinegar Toner, 22
At-Home Microdermabrasion, 70
Aura Glow Highlighter, 59
avocado: about, 178
  Avocado-Aloe Shampoo, 81

Avocado-Coconut Reparative Hair Mask, 100
Avocado-Honey Revitalizing Hair Treatment, 89
Carrot-Avocado Anti-Aging Mask, 41
Revitalizing Cucumber-Avocado Mask, 33

Baking Soda Mask, Anti-Acne, 49
Baking Soda Rinse, Clarifying, 105
Balancing Face Oil, 43
banana: about, 93
  Banana-Honey Dry Scalp Treatment, 87
  Oil-Reducing Banana Mask, 48
  Strengthening Banana Hair Mask, 92
baths and soaks
  Chamomile-Mint Bath Soak, 160–61
  Dead Skin–Dissolving Foot Treatment, 158
  Detoxifying Rosemary Foot Soak, 157
  Ginger-Lemon Oxygen Bath, 155
  Impurity-Dissolving Body Soak, 154
  Indulgent Chocolate Bath, 170
  Invigorating Matcha–Green Tea Bath Soak, 153
  Olive Oil and Rose Bath Soak, 136
  Red Wine Antioxidant Bath, 158–59
  Soothing Oatmeal Bath, 150
Beach Waves Spray, Coconut–Sea Salt, 115
beauty products and ingredients
  apple cider vinegar, 6, 109
  banana, 93

carrier oils, 178–80
commercial brands, 182
essential oils, 177–78
gift packaging, 180–82
honey, 6–7, 88
icon key to recipes, xiii
ingredient sources and specifics, 5–7
lavender, 142, 177
lemon, 66, 177
oatmeal, 151
olive oil, 6, 174, 179–80
pineapple, 45
tea tree oil, 7, 76, 178
tools and utensils for, 8–9
vitamin E oil, 17
yogurt, 6, 53
Beet Lip Stain, 62
Berry-Tinted Lip Balm, 72
Blackhead Eraser, Lemon and Honey, 51
Black Tea Rinse for Deepening Brunette
    Hair, 116
Black Tea Shampoo, Depth-
    Enhancing, 79
blemish and discoloration lighteners
    Acne Scar Eraser, 55
    Anti-Aging Pumpkin Puree Mask, 46
    Apple Cider Vinegar Toner, 22
    At-Home Microdermabrasion, 70
    Brightening and Exfoliating
        Strawberry Mask, 27
    Brightening Citrus Toner, 24
    Carrot-Avocado Anti-Aging Mask, 41
    Dark Circle–Lightening Peach
        Treatment, 61
    Lemon and Honey Blackhead
        Eraser, 51
    Lemon-Yogurt Dark Spot–Lightening
        Treatment, 54
    Olive Oil Skin Salve, 144
    Soothing Chamomile and Oatmeal Face
        Treatment, 36
    Soothing Lavender Eye Balm, 42
    Strawberry Teeth Whitener, 64
    Supergreen Detox Smoothie Facial, 47
    Tea Tree Zit Eraser, 50
Blueberry-Yogurt Mask, Detoxifying, 52
Blush, Hibiscus Glow, 58

body cleansers
    Citrus Salt Scrub, 129
    Foaming Body Wash for Acne-Prone
        Skin, 133
    Honey Body Wash, 128
    Hydrating Coconut Milk Body
        Wash, 127
    Invigorating Coffee Scrub, 134
    Orange-Ginger Foot Scrub, 132
    Pit-Conditioning Deodorant, 130
    Strawberry Body Exfoliant, 131
body detoxifyers
    Anti-Cellulite Ginger Scrub, 159
    Dead Skin–Dissolving Foot
        Treatment, 158
    Detoxifying Mud Body Mask, 156
    Detoxifying Rosemary Foot Soak, 157
    Ginger-Lemon Oxygen Bath, 155
    Impurity-Dissolving Body Soak, 154
    Invigorating Matcha–Green Tea Bath
        Soak, 153
    Red Wine Antioxidant Bath, 158–59
Body-Glow Oil, 146
body moisturizers
    Almond-Rose Body Lotion, 139
    Body-Glow Oil, 146
    Brown Sugar–Vanilla Body Scrub, 152
    Coconut-Lemon-Sugar Body Scrub, 148
    Coconut-Shea Sunscreen, 147
    Homemade Lotion Bars, 145
    Hydrating Body Oil, 137
    Hydrating Coconut Milk Body Wash, 127
    Lavender Hand Cream, 141
    Lemon Cuticle Cream, 149
    Mango Body Butter, 135–36
    Olive Oil and Rose Bath Soak, 136
    Olive Oil Skin Salve, 144
    Peppermint-Vanilla Foot Cream, 143
    Skin-Smoothing Shaving Cream, 138
    Soothing Lavender-Eucalyptus
        Massage Oil, 140
    Soothing Oatmeal Bath, 150
body pampering treatments
    After-Sun Aloe Treatment, 168
    Body Powder, 171
    Chamomile-Mint Bath Soak, 160–61
    Cooling Anti-Itch Treatment, 166

body pampering treatments (*cont.*)
Custom-Blended Perfume, 172
Eucalyptus Bug-Repellent Spray, 167
Indulgent Chocolate Bath, 170
Lavender Hand Cream, 141
Mint-Aloe Cooling Foot Spray, 175
Muscle-Healing Salt Scrub, 161
Olive Oil and Lemon Nail
Strengthener, 173
Olive Oil and Rose Bath Soak, 136
Orange-Ginger Foot Scrub, 132
Peppermint Lotion for Soothing Sore
Muscles, 164
Peppermint–Tea Tree Invigorating
Foot Soak, 162
Rose-Grapefruit Body Spray, 163
Soothing Summer Body Spray, 165
Tea Tree Oil Razor Burn Treatment, 169
Body Powder, 171
Brightening and Exfoliating Strawberry
Mask, 27
Brightening Citrus Toner, 24
Brightening Lemon Cleanser, 30
Bronzing Powder, All-Natural, 67
Brown Sugar Exfoliating Scalp
Treatment, 102
Brown Sugar–Vanilla Body Scrub, 152
Bug-Repellent Spray, Eucalyptus, 167

carrier oils, 178–80
Carrot-Avocado Anti-Aging Mask, 41
Carrot Hair Treatment, Detoxifying, 103
cellulite treatment (Anti-Cellulite Ginger
Scrub), 159
chamomile
Chamomile-Mint Bath Soak, 160–61
Highlight-Enhancing Chamomile
Shampoo, 78
Lemon-Chamomile Lightening Rinse, 117
Soothing Chamomile and Oatmeal Face
Treatment, 36
chocolate
Indulgent Chocolate Bath, 170
Oatmeal-Chocolate Exfoliating Face
Treatment, 28
citrus. *See* lemon; orange
Clarifying Baking Soda Rinse, 105

Clarifying Shampoo, Olive Oil–Lemon, 82
clay masks
Detoxifying Clay Mask, 56
Detoxifying Mud Body Mask, 156
Volumizing Clay Hair Mask, 124
cleansers. *See* body cleansers; facial
cleansers and toners; shampoos
clogged pores. *See* pore decongestants
cocoa butter
Honey–Cocoa Butter Lip Balm, 38
Shea and Cocoa Butter Intense
Hydrating Face Cream, 35
coconut: about, 6, 179
Avocado-Coconut Reparative Hair
Mask, 100
Coconut-Lavender Conditioner, 83
Coconut-Lavender Shampoo, 80
Coconut-Lemon-Sugar Body Scrub, 148
Coconut-Mango Lip Gloss, 68
Coconut–Sea Salt Beach Waves
Spray, 115
Coconut-Shea Sunscreen, 147
Coconut Shine Serum, 98
Coconut–Tea Tree Miracle Scalp
Treatment, 110
Hydrating Coconut Milk Body
Wash, 127
Coffee Conditioning Rinse, Invigorating, 90
Coffee Scrub, Invigorating, 134
conditioners
Coconut-Lavender Conditioner, 83
Conditioning Styling Hair Pomade, 96
Frizz-Taming Hair Serum, 99
Invigorating Coffee Conditioning
Rinse, 90
Cooling Anti-Itch Treatment, 166
Cooling Mint Face Spray, 63
Creamsicle Mask, Orange, 31
cucumber
Cucumber–Olive Oil After-Pool Hair
Revitalizer, 111
De-Puffing Cucumber-Aloe Eye Gel, 60
Refreshing Cucumber Toner, 26
Revitalizing Cucumber-Avocado
Mask, 33
Custom-Blended Perfume, 172
Cuticle Cream, Lemon, 149

Damage-Healing Shine Serum, 118
Dandruff Shampoo, Tea Tree–Jojoba, 75
Dark Circle–Lightening Peach
    Treatment, 61
dark spots. See blemish and discoloration
    lighteners
Dead Skin–Dissolving Foot
    Treatment, 158
deodorants
    Mint-Aloe Cooling Foot Spray, 175
    Pit-Conditioning Deodorant, 130
Depth-Enhancing Black Tea Shampoo, 79
De-Puffing Cucumber-Aloe Eye Gel, 60
Detangling Spray, All-Natural, 123
detoxifying treatments. See body
    detoxifyers; facial detoxifyers; hair
    detoxifyers
discoloration. See blemish and
    discoloration lighteners
dry hair
    Avocado-Aloe Shampoo, 81
    Avocado-Coconut Reparative Hair
        Mask, 100
    Avocado-Honey Revitalizing Hair
        Treatment, 89
    Brown Sugar Exfoliating Scalp
        Treatment, 102
    Coconut-Lavender Conditioner, 83
    Coconut-Lavender Shampoo, 80
    Damage-Healing Shine Serum, 118
    De-Frizzing Hair Rinse, 101
    Depth-Enhancing Black Tea
        Shampoo, 79
    Frizz-Taming Hair Serum, 99
    Highlight-Enhancing Chamomile
        Shampoo, 78
    Hydrating Rose Water Hair Mist, 86
    Invigorating Coffee Conditioning
        Rinse, 90
    Protein-Enriching Hair
        Treatment, 94
    Shea Butter Hair Treatment, 84
    Split End–Mending Balm, 121
    Strengthening Banana Hair Mask, 92
Dry Shampoo, All-Natural, 77
dry skin
    Almond-Rose Body Lotion, 139

Anti-Aging Pumpkin Puree Mask, 46
Balancing Face Oil, 43
Brown Sugar–Vanilla Body Scrub, 152
Hydrating Body Oil, 137
Lemon-Sugar Face Scrub, 65
Mango Body Butter, 135–36
Oatmeal-Chocolate Exfoliating Face
    Treatment, 28
Olive Oil and Honey Mask, 32
Olive Oil Skin Salve, 144
Personalized Facial Cleansing Oil,
    18–19
Shea and Cocoa Butter Intense
    Hydrating Face Cream, 35
Soothing Lavender Eye Balm, 42
Soothing Lavender–Rose Water
    Toner, 20
Soothing Oatmeal Bath, 150

Egg White Mask, Skin-Tightening, 39
essential oils, 177–78
eucalyptus
    Eucalyptus Bug-Repellent Spray, 167
    Soothing Lavender-Eucalyptus
        Massage Oil, 140
exfoliants
    Brightening and Exfoliating
        Strawberry Mask, 27
    Brown Sugar Exfoliating Scalp
        Treatment, 102
    Citrus Salt Scrub, 129
    Decongesting Pineapple Treatment, 44
    Exfoliating Papaya Peel, 29
    Firming Peach Mask, 40
    Foaming Body Wash for Acne-Prone
        Skin, 133
    Oatmeal-Chocolate Exfoliating Face
        Treatment, 28
    Soothing Chamomile and Oatmeal Face
        Treatment, 36
    Strawberry Body Exfoliant, 131
    Supergreen Detox Smoothie Facial, 47
eye treatments
    Dark Circle–Lightening Peach
        Treatment, 61
    De-Puffing Cucumber-Aloe Eye Gel, 60
    Lash-Growth Serum, 71

eye treatments (*cont.*)
Olive Oil Eye-Makeup Remover, 16
Soothing Lavender Eye Balm, 42
Supergreen Detox Smoothie Facial, 47

face pampering treatments
All-Natural Bronzing Powder, 67
At-Home Microdermabrasion, 70
Aura Glow Highlighter, 59
Beet Lip Stain, 62
Berry-Tinted Lip Balm, 72
Coconut-Mango Lip Gloss, 68
Cooling Mint Face Spray, 63
Dark Circle–Lightening Peach
Treatment, 61
De-Puffing Cucumber-Aloe Eye Gel, 60
Hibiscus Glow Blush, 58
Lash-Growth Serum, 71
Lemon-Sugar Face Scrub, 65
Mattifying Face Powder, 69
facial cleansers and toners
All-Natural Makeup-Removing Wipes,
15–16
Apple Cider Vinegar Toner, 22
Brightening and Exfoliating
Strawberry Mask, 27
Brightening Citrus Toner, 24
Brightening Lemon Cleanser, 30
Detoxifying Green Tea Toner, 25
Exfoliating Papaya Peel, 29
Oatmeal-Chocolate Exfoliating Face
Treatment, 28
Oatmeal-Yogurt Cleanser, 21
Olive Oil Eye-Makeup Remover, 16
Olive Oil–Rose Makeup-Removing
Cleanser, 14
Personalized Facial Cleansing Oil, 18–19
Refreshing Cucumber Toner, 26
Soothing Lavender–Rose Water Toner, 20
Tea Tree–Basil Anti-Acne Toner, 23
facial detoxifyers
Acne Scar Eraser, 55
Anti-Acne Baking Soda Mask, 49
Anti-Aging Pumpkin Puree Mask, 46
Decongesting Pineapple Treatment, 44
Detoxifying Blueberry-Yogurt Mask, 52
Detoxifying Clay Mask, 56

Detoxifying Green Tea Toner, 25
Detoxifying Herbal Acne Steam, 57
Lemon and Honey Blackhead Eraser, 51
Lemon-Yogurt Dark Spot–Lightening
Treatment, 54
Oil-Reducing Banana Mask, 48
Supergreen Detox Smoothie Facial, 47
Tea Tree Zit Eraser, 50
facial masks
Anti-Acne Baking Soda Mask, 49
Anti-Aging Pumpkin Puree Mask, 46
Brightening and Exfoliating
Strawberry Mask, 27
Carrot-Avocado Anti-Aging Mask, 41
Decongesting Pineapple Treatment, 44
Detoxifying Blueberry-Yogurt
Mask, 52
Detoxifying Clay Mask, 56
Exfoliating Papaya Peel, 29
Firming Peach Mask, 40
Hydrating Watermelon Mask, 34
Oatmeal-Chocolate Exfoliating Face
Treatment, 28
Oatmeal-Yogurt Cleanser, 21
Oil-Reducing Banana Mask, 48
Olive Oil and Honey Mask, 32
Orange Creamsicle Mask, 31
Revitalizing Cucumber-Avocado
Mask, 33
Skin-Tightening Egg White Mask, 39
facial moisturizers
Balancing Face Oil, 43
Carrot-Avocado Anti-Aging Mask, 41
Firming Peach Mask, 40
Honey–Cocoa Butter Lip Balm, 38
Hydrating Watermelon Mask, 34
Lavender Lip Balm, 37
Olive Oil and Honey Mask, 32
Orange Creamsicle Mask, 31
Revitalizing Cucumber-Avocado
Mask, 33
Shea and Cocoa Butter Intense
Hydrating Face Cream, 35
Soothing Chamomile and Oatmeal Face
Treatment, 36
Soothing Lavender Eye Balm, 42
Firming Peach Mask, 40

Foaming Body Wash for Acne-Prone
  Skin, 133
foot treatments
  Dead Skin–Dissolving Foot
    Treatment, 158
  Detoxifying Rosemary Foot Soak, 157
  Mint-Aloe Cooling Foot Spray, 175
  Orange-Ginger Foot Scrub, 132
  Peppermint–Tea Tree Invigorating
    Foot Soak, 162
  Peppermint-Vanilla Foot Cream, 143
frizzy hair treatments
  Aloe-Almond De-Frizzing Spray, 122
  De-Frizzing Hair Rinse, 101
  Frizz-Taming Hair Serum, 99
  Shea Butter Hair Treatment, 84

gift packaging, 180–82
gifts
  Almond-Rose Body Lotion, 139
  Aura Glow Highlighter, 59
  Beet Lip Stain, 62
  Berry-Tinted Lip Balm, 72
  Body-Glow Oil, 146
  Body Powder, 171
  Brown Sugar–Vanilla Body Scrub, 152
  Chamomile-Mint Bath Soak, 160–61
  Citrus Salt Scrub, 129
  Coconut-Mango Lip Gloss, 68
  Coconut–Sea Salt Beach Waves Spray, 115
  Coconut-Shea Sunscreen, 147
  Coconut Shine Serum, 98
  Conditioning Styling Hair Pomade, 96
  Cooling Mint Face Spray, 63
  Custom-Blended Perfume, 172
  Detoxifying Rosemary Foot Soak, 157
  Eucalyptus Bug-Repellent Spray, 167
  Hair Perfume, 119
  Homemade Lotion Bars, 145
  Honey Body Wash, 128
  Honey–Cocoa Butter Lip Balm, 38
  Hydrating Body Oil, 137
  Hydrating Rose Water Hair Mist, 86
  Lavender Hand Cream, 141
  Lavender Lip Balm, 37
  Lemon Cuticle Cream, 149
  Mint-Aloe Cooling Foot Spray, 175

  Olive Oil Skin Salve, 144
  Orange-Ginger Foot Scrub, 132
  Peppermint Lotion for Soothing Sore
    Muscles, 164
  Peppermint-Vanilla Foot Cream, 143
  Personalized Facial Cleansing Oil,
    18–19
  Rose-Grapefruit Body Spray, 163
  Shea and Cocoa Butter Intense
    Hydrating Face Cream, 35
  Skin-Smoothing Shaving Cream, 138
  Soothing Lavender-Eucalyptus
    Massage Oil, 140
  Soothing Lavender Eye Balm, 42
  Sun-Protection Serum, 114
  Tea Tree Invigorating Scalp Spray, 106
Ginger-Lemon Oxygen Bath, 155
grapefruit
  Invigorating Grapefruit-Mint
    Shampoo, 74–75
  Rose-Grapefruit Body Spray, 163
green tea
  Detoxifying Green Tea Toner, 25
  Invigorating Matcha–Green Tea Bath
    Soak, 153

hair detoxifyers
  Apple Cider Vinegar and Lemon Hair
    Rinse, 108
  Brown Sugar Exfoliating Scalp
    Treatment, 102
  Clarifying Baking Soda Rinse, 105
  Coconut–Tea Tree Miracle Scalp
    Treatment, 110
  Cucumber–Olive Oil After-Pool Hair
    Revitalizer, 111
  Detoxifying Carrot Hair Treatment, 103
  Lemon-Aloe Oil-Reducing Rinse, 104
  Restorative Rosemary-Citrus
    Treatment, 107
  Tea Tree Invigorating Scalp
    Spray, 106
Hair-Growth Serum, 125
hair lighteners
  Coconut–Sea Salt Beach Waves Spray
    (with added lemon), 115
  Hair-Lightening Citrus Mist, 113

hair lighteners (*cont.*)
  Highlight-Enhancing Chamomile
    Shampoo, 78
  Lemon-Chamomile Lightening Rinse, 117
hair moisturizers
  After-Sun Hydrating Hair Treatment, 91
  Avocado-Coconut Reparative Hair
    Mask, 100
  Avocado-Honey Revitalizing Hair
    Treatment, 89
  Banana-Honey Dry Scalp Treatment, 87
  Coconut-Lavender Conditioner, 83
  Coconut Shine Serum, 98
  Conditioning Styling Hair Pomade, 96
  Cucumber–Olive Oil After-Pool Hair
    Revitalizer, 111
  De-Frizzing Hair Rinse, 101
  Frizz-Taming Hair Serum, 99
  Honey-Banana Shine Mask, 97
  Honey Hair Smoothie, 85
  Hydrating Rose Water Hair Mist, 86
  Invigorating Coffee Conditioning
    Rinse, 90
  Protein-Enriching Hair Treatment, 94
  Shea Butter Hair Treatment, 84
  Split End–Banishing Treatment, 95
  Strengthening Banana Hair Mask, 92
hair pampering treatments
  All-Natural Detangling Spray, 123
  All-Natural Hair Spray, 112
  Aloe-Almond De-Frizzing Spray, 122
  Black Tea Rinse for Deepening
    Brunette Hair, 116
  Coconut–Sea Salt Beach Waves
    Spray, 115
  Damage-Healing Shine Serum, 118
  Hair-Growth Serum, 125
  Hair-Lightening Citrus Mist, 113
  Hair Perfume, 119
  Lemon-Chamomile Lightening
    Rinse, 117
  Split End–Mending Balm, 121
  Sun-Protection Serum, 114
  Volumizing Citrus Spray, 120
  Volumizing Clay Hair Mask, 124
hair styling products
  All-Natural Hair Spray, 112

  Coconut–Sea Salt Beach Waves Spray, 115
  Conditioning Styling Hair Pomade, 96
  Volumizing Citrus Spray, 120
hand treatments
  Lavender Hand Cream, 141
  Lemon Cuticle Cream, 149
  Olive Oil and Lemon Nail
    Strengthener, 173
Hibiscus Glow Blush, 58
Highlight-Enhancing Chamomile
  Shampoo, 78
Highlighter, Aura Glow, 59
honey: about, 6–7, 88
  Avocado-Honey Revitalizing Hair
    Treatment, 89
  Banana-Honey Dry Scalp
    Treatment, 87
  Honey-Banana Shine Mask, 97
  Honey Body Wash, 128
  Honey–Cocoa Butter Lip Balm, 38
  Honey Hair Smoothie, 85
  Lemon and Honey Blackhead Eraser, 51
  Olive Oil and Honey Mask, 32
hydration treatments. *See* body
  moisturizers; facial moisturizers;
  hair moisturizers

Impurity-Dissolving Body Soak, 154
Indulgent Chocolate Bath, 170
ingredients. *See* beauty products and
  ingredients
Invigorating Coffee Conditioning Rinse, 90
Invigorating Coffee Scrub, 134
Invigorating Grapefruit-Mint Shampoo,
  74–75
Invigorating Matcha–Green Tea Bath
  Soak, 153

jojoba oil: about, 179
  Tea Tree–Jojoba Dandruff Shampoo, 75

Lash-Growth Serum, 71
lavender: about, 142, 177
  Coconut-Lavender Conditioner, 83
  Coconut-Lavender Shampoo, 80
  Lavender Hand Cream, 141
  Lavender Lip Balm, 37

Soothing Lavender Eye Balm, 42
Soothing Lavender–Rose Water
    Toner, 20
lemon: about, 66, 177
    Brightening Citrus Toner, 24
    Brightening Lemon Cleanser, 30
    Citrus Salt Scrub, 129
    Hair-Lightening Citrus Mist, 113
    Lemon-Aloe Oil-Reducing Rinse, 104
    Lemon and Honey Blackhead Eraser, 51
    Lemon-Chamomile Lightening Rinse, 117
    Lemon Cuticle Cream, 149
    Lemon-Sugar Face Scrub, 65
    Lemon-Yogurt Dark Spot–Lightening
        Treatment, 54
    Mattifying Face Powder, 69
    Restorative Rosemary-Citrus
        Treatment, 107
    Volumizing Citrus Spray, 120
lighteners. See blemish and discoloration
    lighteners; hair lighteners
lip treatments
    Beet Lip Stain, 62
    Berry-Tinted Lip Balm, 72
    Coconut-Mango Lip Gloss, 68
    Honey–Cocoa Butter Lip Balm, 38
    Lavender Lip Balm, 37

makeup
    All-Natural Bronzing Powder, 67
    Aura Glow Highlighter, 59
    Beet Lip Stain, 62
    Berry-Tinted Lip Balm, 72
    Coconut-Mango Lip Gloss, 68
    Hibiscus Glow Blush, 58
    Mattifying Face Powder, 69
makeup removers
    All-Natural Makeup-Removing
        Wipes, 15–16
    Olive Oil Eye-Makeup Remover, 16
    Olive Oil–Rose Makeup-Removing
        Cleanser, 14
mango
    Coconut-Mango Lip Gloss, 68
    Mango Body Butter, 135–36
Massage Oil, Soothing Lavender-
    Eucalyptus, 140

Matcha–Green Tea Bath Soak,
    Invigorating, 153
Mattifying Face Powder, 69
mature skin. See anti-aging treatments
Microdermabrasion, At-Home, 70
mint: about, 178
    Chamomile-Mint Bath Soak, 160–61
    Cooling Mint Face Spray, 63
    Invigorating Grapefruit-Mint
        Shampoo, 74–75
    Mint-Aloe Cooling Foot Spray, 175
    Peppermint Lotion for Soothing Sore
        Muscles, 164
    Peppermint–Tea Tree Invigorating
        Foot Soak, 162
    Peppermint-Vanilla Foot Cream, 143
moisturizers. See body moisturizers; facial
    moisturizers; hair moisturizers
mud masks. See clay masks
Muscle-Healing Salt Scrub, 161
Muscles, Peppermint Lotion for Soothing
    Sore, 164

Nail Strengthener, Olive Oil and Lemon, 173

oatmeal: about, 151
    Oatmeal-Chocolate Exfoliating Face
        Treatment, 28
    Oatmeal-Yogurt Cleanser, 21
    Soothing Chamomile and Oatmeal Face
        Treatment, 36
    Soothing Oatmeal Bath, 150
oils, essential and carrier, 177–80
oily and acne-prone skin
    Acne Scar Eraser, 55
    Anti-Acne Baking Soda Mask, 49
    Apple Cider Vinegar Toner, 22
    Balancing Face Oil, 43
    Brightening Citrus Toner, 24
    Brightening Lemon Cleanser, 30
    Decongesting Pineapple Treatment, 44
    Detoxifying Clay Mask, 56
    Detoxifying Green Tea Toner, 25
    Detoxifying Herbal Acne Steam, 57
    Foaming Body Wash for Acne-Prone
        Skin, 133
    Lemon-Sugar Face Scrub, 65

oily and acne-prone skin (*cont.*)
  Oil-Reducing Banana Mask, 48
  Personalized Facial Cleansing
    Oil, 18–19
  Tea Tree–Basil Anti-Acne Toner, 23
  Tea Tree Zit Eraser, 50
oily hair
  Apple Cider Vinegar and Lemon Hair
    Rinse, 108
  Detoxifying Carrot Hair Treatment, 103
  Invigorating Grapefruit-Mint
    Shampoo, 74–75
  Lemon-Aloe Oil-Reducing Rinse, 104
  Olive Oil–Lemon Clarifying
    Shampoo, 82
  Volumizing Citrus Spray, 120
olive oil: about, 6, 174, 179–80
  Cucumber–Olive Oil After-Pool Hair
    Revitalizer, 111
  Olive Oil and Honey Mask, 32
  Olive Oil and Lemon Nail
    Strengthener, 173
  Olive Oil and Rose Bath Soak, 136
  Olive Oil Eye-Makeup Remover, 16
  Olive Oil–Lemon Clarifying Shampoo, 82
  Olive Oil–Rose Makeup-Removing
    Cleanser, 14
  Olive Oil Skin Salve, 144
orange
  Brightening Citrus Toner, 24
  Orange Creamsicle Mask, 31
  Orange-Ginger Foot Scrub, 132
  Restorative Rosemary-Citrus
    Treatment, 107
  Volumizing Citrus Spray, 120
Oxygen Bath, Ginger-Lemon, 155

pampering treatments. *See* body
  pampering treatments; face pampering
  treatments; gifts; hair pampering
  treatments
Papaya Peel, Exfoliating, 29
Peach Mask, Firming, 40
Peach Treatment, Dark Circle–
  Lightening, 61
peels. *See* exfoliants
peppermint. *See* mint

Perfume, Custom-Blended, 172
Perfume, Hair, 119
Personalized Facial Cleansing Oil, 18–19
pineapple, about, 45
Pineapple Treatment, Decongesting, 44
Pit-Conditioning Deodorant, 130
Pomade, Conditioning Styling Hair, 96
pore decongestants
  Anti-Acne Baking Soda Mask, 49
  Brightening Lemon Cleanser, 30
  Decongesting Pineapple Treatment, 44
  Detoxifying Clay Mask, 56
  Detoxifying Green Tea Toner, 25
  Detoxifying Mud Body Mask, 156
  Firming Peach Mask, 40
  Lemon and Honey Blackhead Eraser, 51
Protein-Enriching Hair Treatment, 94
Pumpkin Puree Mask, Anti-Aging, 46

Razor Burn Treatment, Tea Tree Oil, 169
Red Wine Antioxidant Bath, 158–59
Refreshing Cucumber Toner, 26
Restorative Rosemary-Citrus
  Treatment, 107
Revitalizing Cucumber-Avocado Mask, 33
rose: about, 178
  Almond-Rose Body Lotion, 139
  Hydrating Rose Water Hair Mist, 86
  Olive Oil and Rose Bath Soak, 136
  Olive Oil–Rose Makeup-Removing
    Cleanser, 14
  Soothing Lavender–Rose Water
    Toner, 20
Rose-Grapefruit Body Spray, 163
Rosemary-Citrus Treatment,
  Restorative, 107
Rosemary Foot Soak, Detoxifying, 157

scars. *See* blemish and discoloration
  lighteners
scrubs
  Anti-Cellulite Ginger Scrub, 159
  Brown Sugar–Vanilla Body Scrub, 152
  Citrus Salt Scrub, 129
  Coconut-Lemon-Sugar Body
    Scrub, 148
  Invigorating Coffee Scrub, 134

Lemon-Sugar Face Scrub, 65
Muscle-Healing Salt Scrub, 161
Orange-Ginger Foot Scrub, 132
shampoos
All-Natural Dry Shampoo, 77
Avocado-Aloe Shampoo, 81
Coconut-Lavender Shampoo, 80
Depth-Enhancing Black Tea
Shampoo, 79
Highlight-Enhancing Chamomile
Shampoo, 78
Invigorating Grapefruit-Mint
Shampoo, 74–75
Olive Oil–Lemon Clarifying
Shampoo, 82
Tea Tree–Jojoba Dandruff Shampoo, 75
Shaving Cream, Skin-Smoothing, 138
shea butter
Coconut-Shea Sunscreen, 147
Shea and Cocoa Butter Intense
Hydrating Face Cream, 35
Shea Butter Hair Treatment, 84
skin care, facial. *See entries beginning
with* facial
skin irritation
Cooling Anti-Itch Treatment, 166
Olive Oil Skin Salve, 144
Soothing Oatmeal Bath, 150
Soothing Summer Body Spray, 165
Tea Tree Oil Razor Burn
Treatment, 169
Skin-Smoothing Shaving Cream, 138
Skin-Tightening Egg White Mask, 39
Smoothie, Honey Hair, 85
soaks. *See* baths and soaks
Soothing Chamomile and Oatmeal Face
Treatment, 36
Soothing Lavender-Eucalyptus Massage
Oil, 140
Soothing Lavender Eye Balm, 42
Soothing Lavender–Rose Water
Toner, 20
Soothing Oatmeal Bath, 150
Soothing Summer Body Spray, 165
Split End–Banishing Treatment, 95
Split End–Mending Balm, 121
Steam, Detoxifying Herbal Acne, 57

strawberries
Berry-Tinted Lip Balm, 72
Brightening and Exfoliating
Strawberry Mask, 27
Strawberry Body Exfoliant, 131
Strawberry Teeth Whitener, 64
sun exposure
After-Sun Aloe Treatment, 168
After-Sun Hydrating Hair
Treatment, 91
Avocado-Aloe Shampoo, 81
Coconut-Shea Sunscreen, 147
Sun-Protection Serum, 114
Supergreen Detox Smoothie
Facial, 47

tea tree oil: about, 7, 76, 178
Coconut–Tea Tree Miracle Scalp
Treatment, 110
Peppermint–Tea Tree Invigorating
Foot Soak, 162
Tea Tree–Basil Anti-Acne Toner, 23
Tea Tree Invigorating Scalp
Spray, 106
Tea Tree–Jojoba Dandruff
Shampoo, 75
Tea Tree Oil Razor Burn
Treatment, 169
Tea Tree Zit Eraser, 50
Teeth Whitener, Strawberry, 64
toners. *See* facial cleansers and toners

vitamin E oil, about, 17
Volumizing Citrus Spray, 120
Volumizing Clay Hair Mask, 124

washes. *See* body cleansers
Watermelon Mask, Hydrating, 34

yogurt: about, 6, 53
Detoxifying Blueberry-Yogurt
Mask, 52
Lemon-Yogurt Dark Spot–Lightening
Treatment, 54
Oatmeal-Yogurt Cleanser, 21

Zit Eraser, Tea Tree, 50

About the Author

ANNIE STROLE is a makeup artist, natural-beauty expert and contributing editor for style, beauty and DIY site Lovelyish.com.

Born and raised in Texas, Annie now lives in Brooklyn with her cat, dog, husband and son. This is her first book.